Contemporary Issues in Occupational Therapy

Reasoning and Reflection

Contemporary Issues in Occupational Therapy

Reasoning and Reflection

Edited by

JENNIFER CREEK AND ANNE LAWSON-PORTER

BICENTENNIAL
1807
WILEY
2007
BICENTENNIAL

John Wiley & Sons, Ltd

MT

Copyright © 2007   John Wiley & Sons Ltd
                       The Atrium, Southern Gate, Chichester,
                       West Sussex PO19 8SQ, England
                       Telephone   (+44) 1243 779777

Email (for orders and customer service enquiries): cs-books@wiley.co.uk
Visit our Home Page on www.wiley.com

Other Wiley Editorial Offices

John Wiley & Sons Inc., 111 River Street, Hoboken, NJ 07030, USA

Jossey-Bass, 989 Market Street, San Francisco, CA 94103-1741, USA

Wiley-VCH Verlag GmbH, Boschstr. 12, D-69469 Weinheim, Germany

John Wiley & Sons Australia Ltd, 42 McDougall Street, Milton, Queensland 4064, Australia

John Wiley & Sons (Asia) Pte Ltd, 2 Clementi Loop #02-01, Jin Xing Distripark, Singapore 129809

John Wily & Sons Canada Ltd, 6045 Freemont Blvd, Mississauga, ONT, L5R 4J3.

Wiley also publishes its books in a variety of electronic formats. Some content that appears in print may not be available in electronic books.

Anniversary Logo Design: Richard J. Pacifico

Library of Congress Cataloging-in-Publication Data

Contemporary issues in occupational therapy : reasoning and reflection / edited by Jennifer Creek and Anne Lawson-Porter. – 2nd ed.
     p.   ;   cm.
    Includes bibliographical references and index.
    ISBN 978-0-470-06511-2 (pbk. : alk. paper)   1. Occupational therapy.   2. Outcome assessment (Medical care)   I. Creek, Jennifer.   II. Lawson-Porter, Anne.
    [DNLM: 1. Occupational Therapy–trends.   WB 555 C761 2007]
    RM735.C66357 2007
    615.8'515–dc22

                                                                    2006102034

A catalogue record for this book is available from the British Library

ISBN 978-0-470-06511-2

Typeset by SNP Best-set Typesetter Ltd, Hong Kong
Printed and bound in Great Britain by TJ International Ltd, Padstow, Cornwall

This book is printed on acid-free paper responsibly manufactured from sustainable forestry in which at least two trees are planted for each one used for paper production.

2\1\08

Contents

About the editors

Jennifer Creek has been an occupational therapist since 1970, when she qualified from the London School of Occupational Therapy. She has worked in the fields of adult mental health, adult learning disabilities, mental health promotion and occupational therapy education. She is the editor of a textbook *Occupational Therapy and Mental Health*, which is about to go into its fourth edition. This is her second edited collection of essays. She is currently working with the European Network of Occupational Therapists in Higher Education terminology project group to produce a conceptual framework for occupational therapy in Europe.

Anne Lawson-Porter qualified as an occupational therapist in 1974 and worked in the field of physical dysfunction for the first ten years of her career in both health and social care settings. Her next move was into occupational therapy education; she has taught occupational therapists at both undergraduate and post-graduate levels. Her passion for occupational therapy was renewed in the move to her current post as Head of Education for the College of Occupational Therapists where she continues to work hard to influence and develop learning opportunities for all members of the profession.

Contributors

Katrina Bannigan BD, BSc, PhD, PgCLTHE
Faculty of Health and Life Sciences, York St John University, Lord Mayor's Walk, York, UK

Rosemary F. Caulton NZOTR, BSc (Econ), Post Grad Cert Ed, MA (Anthropology)
School of Occupational Therapy, Otago Polytechnic, Dunedin, New Zealand

Jennifer Creek FCOT, MSc, DipCOT, FETC
Freelance Occupational Therapist, Guisborough, North Yorkshire, UK

Rayna D. Dickson NZOTR, BSc (Occupational Therapy), Cert Community Psychiatric Care (University of Otago), Dip Teaching (Tertiary), Post Grad Dip Arts (Anthropology/Education), MA (Anthropology)
School of Occupational Therapy, Otago Polytechnic, Dunedin, New Zealand

Priscilla Harries PhD, MSc, DipCOT, MILT
Course Leader, MSc Occupational Therapy, Mary Seacole Building, Brunel University, Uxbridge, London, UK

Clare Hocking PhD, MHSc(OT)
AUT University, Auckland, New Zealand

Anne Lawson-Porter MEd, DipCOT
Group Head of Education, College of Occupational Therapists, London, UK

Lindsey Nicholls MA, BSc
Department of Occupational Therapy, Faculty Community and Health Sciences, University Western Cape, Bellville, South Africa

Ellen Nicholson MOcc Therapy
Professional Potential Ltd, Auckland, New Zealand

Kit Sinclair PhD, MPHE, BScOT
Department of Rehabilitation Sciences, Hong Kong Polytechnic University, Hung Hom, Hong Kong, China

Elizabeth White PhD, DipCOT
Head of Research and Development, College of Occupational Therapists, London, UK

Foreword

Elizabeth White

Occupational therapy is a profession that has been in existence for 90 years. During its lifetime there have been major changes in the predominant diseases that affect people worldwide and lead to the need for therapeutic interventions. Accompanying this have been significant demographic alterations, immense developments in societal structures and expectations and an enormous increase in the availability and delivery of health and social care. Against this background, the notion of publishing a book entitled *Contemporary Issues in Occupational Therapy* may seem to pose a mammoth task.

Creek and Lawson-Porter have approached this task by producing an international collection of essays with a focus on reasoning and reflection. Their selected authors present a range of perspectives that demonstrate how reflection on clinical experiences has shaped their own professional development. By use of case-study illustrations and carefully selected quotations, it can be seen that maintaining a focus on meaningful occupations is central to professional practice, allowing the therapist to work with individual service users to bring physical, mental and social well-being as well as societal gain.

Through the initial chapters of the book, the focus is on the common theme of theoretical and philosophical tenets of occupational therapy and how these influence, and are influenced by, the thinking and reasoning activities of occupational therapists. The following chapters shift the emphasis to the practice of occupational therapy. The complexity of reasoning which supports an expert therapist's actions is seen as a key skill of professional practice. By reflecting on interactions with service users within the environments in which they live their lives, and using this knowledge to shape future interventions, occupational therapists can grow an understanding about their own capacity and skills.

In 2006, Nixon and Creek posed two questions for the profession: 'what characterizes professional practice and how does thoughtfulness relate to occupational therapy practice?' (Nixon and Creek, 2006, p. 77). Through the contributions of some of the current expert thinkers in the field of occupational therapy, Creek and Lawson-Porter steer a pathway that offers some deliberation on these questions within an international perspective. In the twenty-first century, it is evident that the resurgence of meaningful occupation as the central focus of the activities of occupational therapists is shaping professional identify and development. Reasoning and reflection allow occupational therapists to develop the language and concepts of occupation that contextualize and inform their own practice, and will drive the profession into its rightful role as a key contributor to the health and well-being of our populations.

Reference

Nixon, J. and Creek, J. (2006) Towards a theory of practice. *British Journal of Occupational Therapy* **69**(2), 77–80.

Preface

Ten years ago, Jennifer became enthused by a new energy and confidence within the profession of occupational therapy that was apparent in conference papers, journal articles and other publications. After talking with colleagues, she decided to try to capture some of these developments by inviting people whose work she most respected to write extended essays on their chosen subjects. The aim was to give them a chance to expound their ideas in some depth, in the hope of provoking more critical debate within the profession. Colin Whurr (publisher) expressed an interest in the project and the result was a collection of nine essays on aspects of theory and practice: *Occupational Therapy: New Perspectives*.

Jennifer and Anne worked together about fifteen years ago, whereupon Anne became enthused by Jennifer's theoretical approach to explaining what occupational therapists do and why. That fascination has continued to recent times and when an opportunity arose to work collaboratively in the editing of this new edition it was an opportunity not to be passed over. The journey of further exploration has been educational, enlightening and inspirational; all fed by some wonderful theorists and writers in occupational therapy.

Over the past decade, there have been many exciting new developments in the theory and practice of occupational therapy, such as an increased awareness of the political aspects of disease and disability and an emerging role for occupational therapists in health promotion and community development. Much of this energy comes from countries where occupational therapy is a relative newcomer to the health-care scene or where the problems are so overwhelming that therapists are having to find new ways of working. The changing nature of occupational therapy is being mapped in a succession of textbooks and other publications that are enriching the professional literature base.

One of the theoretical developments that has captured our imaginations in recent years is the adoption by occupational therapists of complexity theory as a way of understanding the relationships between people, occupation and health. Occupational therapists are developing their thinking skills in order to work with the full complexity of these relationships. A complex intervention requires the therapist to make many judgements and decisions throughout the process, weighing up many factors in order to take the most appropriate course of action.

We are indebted to many people, but particularly to Sarah Cook, Elizabeth White and Jon Nixon for the long discussions we have had about the importance of thinking to occupational therapy practice. These discussions helped to give shape to this collection of essays, which focuses on the different ways that therapists think and how they use their thinking skills in practice.

Jennifer Creek and Anne Lawson-Porter

Acknowledgements

The editors would like to thank all those occupational therapists, students and service users who have been the inspiration for the contributors to this book. Special thanks go to those particular colleagues who have shared thoughts and been willing to explore issues, with the common goal of developing thinking and practice in occupational therapy.

Introduction

Jennifer Creek and Anne Lawson-Porter

At the beginning of the twenty-first century, the profession of occupational therapy is undergoing radical changes that will determine the direction in which it develops during the next few decades. This quiet revolution marks a shift from systems thinking, which has guided occupational therapy theory and practice for over 40 years, to complexity thinking.

Over thirty years ago, the influential American occupational therapist, Mary Reilly, suggested that the profession should develop a general theory of occupational therapy, using general systems theory as an organising framework (Reilly, 1974). General systems theory is a way of understanding the relationships between elements in the material world that is hierarchical in organization. Elements are categorized at different levels of complexity, with each level subordinate to the ones above and incorporating the ones below. For example, atoms are made up of protons and electrons, molecules are made of atoms, cells are made of molecules, men are made of cells and social organisations are made of men (Boulding, 1968).

General systems theory has provided a coherent structure for the development of many models for occupational therapy practice, but ways of making sense of the world change. In 1962, the American philosopher of science, Thomas Kuhn, wrote a book, *The Structure of Scientific Revolutions*, in which he demonstrated that the way knowledge develops in society is through revolutions rather than incremental changes.

Kuhn said that the body of knowledge created by a scientific community represents their world view, or *paradigm*. The paradigm of the community supplies the foundation for practice and attracts a group of adherents away from competing paradigms. For example, people who choose to be occupational therapists espouse the beliefs, theories and practices of occupational therapy rather than those of nursing or psychology. Kuhn said that having a paradigm transforms a group into a profession or, at least, into a discipline.

During a period of what Kuhn called *normal science*, there is a dominant accepted paradigm and general agreement about the nature of things within the community. Fundamental novelties and competing world views are suppressed, ignored or ridiculed because they are necessarily subversive of the basic beliefs and commitments of the scientific community. However, as knowledge accumulates, there are more and more challenges to the current paradigm. Eventually, there is a revolution in which one of the competing paradigms becomes generally accepted, and a new period of normal science commences.

General systems theory provided occupational therapy with hierarchical structures that have been used to organise the knowledge generated by research and scholarly activity over several decades, but the challenges to this way of seeing the world have become too numerous and persistent to ignore. These challenges come from demographic changes, leading to changing patterns of need, as well as from new theoretical influences and research findings.

One of the theories gaining ground in occupational therapy, as well as in many other disciplines, is complexity. This theory attempts to understand 'the irregular, unpredictable behaviour of deterministic, nonlinear dynamic systems' (Gleick, 1987, p. 306). It accepts unpredictability and does not demand that complex phenomena should be simplified or controlled in order to be understood. Relationships and interactions between components in a complex system are non-linear, which means that the system cannot be described or understood in terms of its components. A system with a large number of components that interact in a linear fashion is complicated, not complex.

In 2003, the College of Occupational Therapists published a definition of occupational therapy as a complex intervention (Creek, 2003). This document describes occupational therapy as 'a partnership between the therapist and client in which both participate actively' (p. 8). In order for the therapist to be able to recognise and work with all the elements involved in client-centred practice – the goals and processes of intervention; the client's needs and wishes, and the social, political and working contexts – it is necessary to use a range of thinking skills. At each stage of the occupational therapy process, the therapist uses types of thinking appropriate to the issues being considered. These thinking skills include analysis, reasoning and reflection.

Since the 1980s, several studies have been carried out into the types of thinking that underpin the practice of highly skilled professionals. In 1982, Patricia Benner published a study of how nurses develop from novice to expert practitioners (Benner, 1982). A year later, Donald Schön published *The Reflective Practitioner*, which looked at how professionals think in action (Schön, 1983). In the 1990s, the American Occupational Therapy Association funded a study of clinical reasoning that identified how therapists move between different modes of reasoning as they interact with their clients (Mattingly and Fleming, 1994). All these publications have encouraged occupational therapists to recognise the complexity of their work and to feel confident in their thinking skills.

This collection of essays represents the work of ten occupational therapy theorists from around the world, all of whom have embraced the challenge of complexity. The first essay, 'The thinking therapist' by Jennifer Creek, sets the theme of the book. This thoughtful exposition reminds us of the core skills of the occupational therapist and explores three approaches to practice; technician, technologist, thinker, and their manifestation as novices to experts, before acknowledging that a combination of all three approaches is needed in expert occupational therapy practice. This chapter will provide readers with the thinking needed to capitalise on the themes in the rest of this book.

Clare Hocking explores Romantic assumptions about the power of arts and crafts to bring about change from illness and despair to hope and self-respect. Her essay captures the sense of excitement and triumph felt by the first occupational therapists as they saw their patients transformed by their engagement in creative activities. These practitioners clearly saw themselves restoring people's lives, not just their health. Much of this passion and confidence has been lost to the profession but Clare demonstrates that some Romantic notions still survive.

In 'Occupation for occupational therapists', Clare Hocking and Ellen Nicholson tackle two controversial topics: occupation as the exclusive domain of occupational therapists and whether specialists in particular fields of practice are still occupational therapists. They ask difficult questions such as should we willingly share our knowledge with others and does embracing a specialism mean giving up a concern with occupation? No easy answers are offered, but the authors highlight the need for further reflection and debate within the profession.

Lindsey Nichols takes as her starting point the observation that occupational therapists have cast off part of their theoretical heritage and, in doing so, have lost some of the richness of the profession. She argues that psychoanalytic theory, with its appreciation of the role that the unconscious mind plays in shaping what we do, provides an invaluable tool for therapists to reach a more informed understanding of their own reasons for what they do, as well as the motivations of their clients.

Rosemary Caulton and Rayna Dickson explore the nature of knowing, showing and telling in occupational therapy education and practice, through community-based practice placements where activity and community integration, and services to support them, are the objectives. The authors describe how practitioners focus on the services that they are providing rather than on the articulation of what they are doing and why. They go on to explore how they use their observations of students and educators in practice, through further exploration of occupational and anthropological literature, to form a coherent body of knowledge that informs the nature of occupation within cultures, the role of the practitioner and the use of literature in understanding practice.

Liz White describes the difficulties faced by occupational therapists when prescribing wheelchairs for people with severe disabilities. The essay builds a picture of the many interacting elements that the therapist has to incorporate into her clinical reasoning, and shows how paying attention to the needs of carers can seem incompatible with meeting the needs of the disabled wheelchair user. We are given a graphic illustration of the complexity of occupational therapy practice.

If occupational therapy is to be a true partnership between the therapist and client, it is necessary for the client to feel fully involved in the process of intervention. Jennifer Creek offers a way of thinking about the client who is hard to engage, and offers some practical suggestions for overcoming problems of motivation, volition or autonomy.

Kit Sinclair has produced an elegant matrix of clinical reasoning skills, building on the work of theorists such as Benner, Mattingly and Fleming. She describes the research methods that she has used in developing the facets of clinical reasoning which are then utilised to develop the Sinclair Matrix. This matrix provides a model that combines the knowledge, skills and experience required to develop clinical reasoning, and Sinclair explores how educators in academia and practice can help students gain competence and expertise in clinical reasoning through a sequential approach.

Priscilla Harries continues the theme of developing competence in students, this time in relation to the prioritisation of referrals through wise clinical judgements. Her research explores how clinicians in community mental health teams make judgements. The role that reflection has in refining and developing wisdom and its impact on managing case loads to the benefit of users and services is further explored before culminating in a strategy to enable students to develop the ability to make wise judgements in readiness for professional practice.

There is an expanding body of research into how research findings influence practice. Katrina Bannigan explores how difficult it can be to disseminate research findings in ways that will lead to positive changes in clinical practice. She offers systems thinking as a way of making sense of research utilisation, but warns that there is still a long way to go in reducing the research–practice gap in occupational therapy.

The essays in this volume cover theory, practice and research in occupational therapy. They explore professional reasoning and reflection in ways that are in full measure fascinating and challenging. Reading them will take you on a journey through the world of thinking that will allow you to explore your own thinking in relation to each of the topics, with the expectation that your new thinking will improve your own theoretical approaches to your work, in ways that will benefit the people who use your services.

References

Benner, P. (1982) From novice to expert. *American Journal of Nursing*, **82**, 402–7.
Boulding, K.E. (1968) General systems theory – the skeleton of science, in *Modern Systems Research for the Behavioural Scientist* (ed. W. Buckley), Aldine, Chicago, pp. 3–10.

Creek, J. (2003) *Occupational Therapy Defined as a Complex Intervention*. College of Occupational Therapists, London.

Gleick, J. (1987) *Chaos: Making a New Science*. Abacus, London.

Kuhn, T. (1962) *The Structure of Scientific Revolutions*. University of Chicago Press, Chicago.

Mattingly, C. and Fleming, M.H. (1994) *Clinical Reasoning: Forms of Inquiry in a Therapeutic Practice*. FA Davis, Philadelphia.

Reilly, M. (1974) An explanation of play, in *Play as Exploratory Learning: Studies of Curiosity Behavior* (ed. M. Reilly). Sage, Beverly Hills, CA, pp. 117–55.

Schön, D.A. (1983) *The Reflective Practitioner: How Professionals Think in Action*. Basic Books, New York.

The thinking therapist

1

Jennifer Creek

Introduction

The practice of occupational therapy had its beginnings in the wards of long-stay psychiatric institutions, with the first occupational therapists providing systematic programmes of purposeful activity for people who were excluded from society and confined. Many of these institutions contained as many as 2000 or more inmates and they were built on the outskirts of towns (Paterson, 2002), providing a visible indication of the marginalised status of the inmates.

Occupational therapists working in these institutions used interesting, soothing and pleasurable activities to occupy the time and hold the interest of patients: 'a program of wholesome living as the *basis* of wholesome feeling and thinking and fancy and interests' (Meyer, 1977, p. 641). Their aim was to enable patients to discover for themselves how engagement in routines of activity could help them to adapt and learn to manage their mental health problems so that they might become reintegrated into society as productive and worthy citizens.

> The purpose of the occupational therapist in treating cases of mental disorder is to provide means for the re-education of those functions of the mind which are either not functioning or are functioning abnormally, i.e.: to train the patient who has lost the power of concentration to concentrate again; to revive lost powers of initiative and to bring the patient who is living in a world of phantasy into touch with real things again; to stimulate and restore confidence in herself in the depressed patient; to engage the mind so that delusions and

hallucinations which distress the patient when her attention is not otherwise held, are for a time driven out.

(Haworth and MacDonald, 1946, p. 10)

This approach to treatment was based on the principle that people have a fundamental need to be active:

Our conception of man is that of an organism that maintains and balances itself in the world of reality and actuality by being in active life and active use, i.e., using and living and acting its *time* in harmony with its own nature and the nature about it.

(Meyer, 1977, p. 641)

Although the way that society treats people with mental illness has changed, so that there is no longer the same need to occupy people during long hospital admissions, occupational therapy practice is still based on the belief that people are intrinsically active and that their health and well-being are influenced by what they do (Creek, 2003). The American occupational therapist, Mary Reilly, expressed this in the well-known phrase: 'that man, through the use of his hands as they are energized by mind and will, can influence the state of his own health' (Reilly, 1962, p. 2). Reilly said that 'a profession organized around this hypothesis sets few limits to its growth' (1962, p. 2), and the development of the profession over the past 100 years has not refuted this claim. Occupational therapy has adapted to changing social, political and economic climates throughout its history and has expanded successfully into different cultures all over the world.

The profession of occupational therapy started in the United States, with a group of interested people from different professional backgrounds meeting in 1917 to establish the National Society for the Promotion of Occupational Therapy (Paterson, 2002, p. 8). The World Federation of Occupational Therapists (WFOT) was established in 1952 when 'a small number of senior members of the profession . . . decided that the increasing growth and strength of the profession warranted and indeed made imperative the establishment of an international body' (Mendez, 1986, p. 1). The first WFOT Council meeting was held in Edinburgh in 1954, attended by 10 founder member countries. At the beginning of the twenty-first century, WFOT has 60 member countries: 52 full members and eight associate members.

The first British occupational therapist trained in the United States and was employed in Scotland in 1928 (Paterson, 2002). Nearly 80 years later, there are over 26,000 occupational therapists registered to practise in the UK (Health Professions Council, n.d.). In the early days, most occupational therapists worked in psychiatric hospitals, general hospitals or social services departments. Now, in the United Kingdom, they work in accident and emergency departments, community settings, forensic units, people's homes and workplaces, primary care clinics, prisons, schools, sheltered housing, in fact, in almost all the places where people live their lives.

This essay discusses the knowledge and skills that an occupational therapist needs in order to practise effectively in all these settings and to fulfil her professional purpose. The first section discusses occupational therapy practice and identifies the core skills of the practitioner. The next section describes three approaches to practice: the practitioner as technician, technologist or thinker. The third section considers the nature of professional expertise and describes the difference between novice and expert technicians, technologists and thinkers. The final section concludes that all three approaches need to be integrated to achieve true expertise in occupational therapy practice.

What does an occupational therapist do?

Human beings have an occupational nature (Wilcock, 1998) therefore, in order to maintain health and well-being, people need to be active and organise their activities into flexible routines that have personal meaning and social value. When someone's ability to engage in activity and to participate in society is impaired by a health condition or by circumstances (World Health Organization, 2001), the occupational therapist assists him to gain, maintain, improve or regain the skills to support everyday life. Occupational therapy has been succinctly described as 'the process of finding creative, appropriate and contextually relevant ways of dealing with those life challenges that create the need for intervention' (Christiansen, 2006, p. xii).

Much of what occupational therapists do is concerned with the tasks and activities of everyday life, which are taken for granted until we cannot perform them because of illness or disability. The goals of intervention can appear commonplace but the approaches used to achieve those goals are sophisticated and highly skilled. Assessment and intervention are tailored to the occupational needs of individuals within the contexts where they expect to live and work (Creek *et al.*, 2005). This means that the occupational therapist must have a broad knowledge base and a wide array of practical skills that can be applied flexibly to suit different problems and circumstances. In addition, she must be able to think carefully and creatively to decide on the best course of action, and that thinking should be a collaborative process with the client and others. Professional judgement is always exercised in a social context and, 'to be effective, must be dialogical' (Nixon and Creek, 2006, p. 78).

The practice of occupational therapy utilises a set of core skills (Creek, 2003):

- Building collaborative relationships with clients that will promote reflection, autonomy and engagement in the therapeutic process;
- Assessing and observing functional potential, limitations, ability and needs, including the effects of physical and psychosocial environments;
- Enabling people to explore, achieve and maintain balance in their occupations in the areas of personal care, domestic life, leisure and productivity;
- Identifying and solving occupational performance problems;
- Promoting health, well-being and function by analysing, selecting, synthesising, adapting, grading and applying activities for specific therapeutic purposes;
- Planning, organising and leading activity groups;
- Analysing and adapting environments to increase function and social participation.

These skills incorporate three elements that interact with each other as the therapist assesses, makes judgements, negotiates, takes action and evaluates the impact of her actions:

1. **Practical skills**: the techniques that the therapist has mastered, which make up a personal toolbox. These skills include communication, interpersonal and teamworking skills, skills and techniques for assessment and therapy, time management and self-management skills.

2. **Knowledge and understanding**: the theories that can be used to describe situations, build an explanation for what is happening and predict the effect of different interventions. The knowledge base of the occupational therapist includes concepts, theories, frames of reference, approaches and models. These may be specific to occupational therapy, such as the classification of occupations (Creek, 2002), or have been developed within other disciplines, such as the social model of disability.

3. **Thinking skills**: the mental actions used by the therapist in framing problems and working out the best solutions. The thinking skills of the occupational therapist include clinical reasoning, decision making, reflection, analysis and ethical reasoning.

Practical skills, knowledge and thinking are necessary elements of the practice of occupational therapy but not all practitioners give them equal weight.

Some occupational therapists put more emphasis on their practical skills; some are more concerned with using theory and models to direct their practice, and some see occupational therapy as a complex intervention that requires them to reflect, make case-by-case judgements and negotiate the most appropriate action to be taken at each point in the process (Creek, 2003).

The way that the therapist works will depend on which of these approaches she is using. For example, the practitioner working in mental health, who bases her practice on technical skills, may organise daily programmes of therapeutic groups to which clients are allocated following an assessment of their needs. The practitioner who uses a single model or frame of reference will apply the same process of assessment with each client and formulate his problems within the framework of that model. The practitioner for whom thinking is central to practice sees the client's mental health problems as part of a wider picture and uses a variety of theories and practical skills to suit particular needs at particular times.

Approaches to occupational therapy practice

The early occupational therapists were skilled practitioners, with knowledge of a wide range of crafts and other activities. They were also expert at communicating with their clients and engaging them in carefully planned programmes of activity that would serve therapeutic purposes. An occupational therapy textbook published in 1955 advised that: 'The Occupational Therapist must have the necessary technical knowledge, special aptitude for imparting instruction, and a suitable temperament and manner' (O'Sullivan, 1955, p. 28).

Fifty years after this was written, occupational therapy practice still requires the practitioner to have a good range of skills and techniques. The student on practice placement learns generic skills, such as communication, observation, reporting and record keeping, and specific practice skills, such as assessment of motor skills, group facilitation or wheelchair prescription. The beginning practitioner usually concentrates on building up a sound repertoire of skills within the area of practice she has chosen. A good therapist will continue to learn new skills and techniques throughout her career, keeping up to date with social, technological and professional developments.

Some occupational therapists are satisfied that having a good range of practical skills enables them to meet the needs of their clients. These therapists often describe their practice in terms of the techniques they use, for example, 'I'm a creative therapist' or 'I supply assistive devices and recommend housing adaptations'. This practitioner is *the technician*.

The technician

A technician is 'a person skilled in the technique or mechanical part of an art or craft' (*Shorter Oxford English Dictionary*, 2002). In occupational therapy, this is the practitioner who has highly developed practical skills, usually in a particular field or approach to practice. For example, the therapist might have expertise in working with amputees or in using projective techniques.

Every occupational therapist learns a range of generic and specialist practical skills, which will continue to expand throughout her career. The experienced therapist will have more skills, at a higher level of competence, than a beginner. Any change of field will necessitate learning a new set of skills and techniques specific to the new area of practice. The technician may be skilled in a few techniques or many. These may be techniques that are applicable across a range of practice areas, for example teaching activities of daily living, or useful mainly within an area of specialisation, such as stress management.

A qualified occupational therapist is expected to have more transferable skills and a wider range of skills than a support worker. A study of the relationship between qualified and unqualified staff in the remedial professions in the 1970s concluded that an experienced unqualified worker is expected to have practical knowledge of the job but not to have the theoretical knowledge that would make their skills transferable (Alaszewski and Meltzer, 1979). This is not the case in some other countries, such as South Africa, where support workers have both a practical and a theoretical education.

Occupational therapy is concerned with what people do and how they do it; therefore much of the profession's value and status comes from practical interventions that make a visible difference in people's lives. However, this does not mean that all occupational therapists practise as technicians: some feel the need to have a more explicit way of understanding the process of change that people go through in adjusting to disease or disability. They seek theories to explain how disease and disability impact on function and indicate what actions might be taken to remediate dysfunction. The practitioner who uses a theoretical framework as a guide for applying knowledge in her daily work is *the technologist* (Christiansen, 2006).

The technologist

In the first half of the twentieth century, occupational therapists worked under the direction of medical staff, making a clear distinction between the use of occupation as therapy and its use for other, non-curative purposes such as earning money (O'Sullivan, 1955). The doctor provided the knowledge of medical theory that enabled occupations to be used therapeutically: the occupational therapist provided the practical skills to engage patients in activity. In effect, the occupational therapist was a technician working under the direction of the doctor.

This relationship continued until the late 1950s, when it became apparent 'that too much emphasis [had] been put upon the diversional and occupational aspects of activities to the neglect of the psychodynamic problems of the individual receiving occupational therapy' (Azima and Wittkower, 1957, p. 1). The authors of a study of occupational therapy in psychiatric hospitals in North America (Azima and Wittkower, 1957) concluded that this was due, in large part, to the lack of a theory of occupational therapy and to the inability of psychiatrists to perform the expected role of authority. The time had come for the profession to develop its own theory base.

In the early 1980s, the American social scientist, Donald Schön (1983), said that the professions do not only have specialist skills, they also hold specialist knowledge and apply it in order to solve the complex and obstinate problems of society. For example, the medical profession applies specialist knowledge to the cure of disease, with the object of producing a healthy society; the economist assumes responsibility for the economic well-being of society through managing the flow of money, and the teacher is the expert in educating the next generation to the standards set by society. Schön suggested that a rapid increase in the number of professions at the beginning of the twentieth century was directly related to a growing social need for technical expertise.

As the amount of scientific knowledge in the world increases, it becomes more and more difficult for any one person to know everything there is to know in his own area of expertise. This has led to narrower specialisation and a separation of the functions of knowledge creation and knowledge application. The task of producing and testing knowledge now belongs to scholars, researchers and academics, who tend to be employed within universities. The application of knowledge is the job of professionals, who are usually employed in practice positions (Schön, 1983).

Within occupational therapy, research and theory development are mostly carried out by the faculty of universities, while the resultant knowledge is applied by occupational therapy practitioners employed in health and social care contexts. This separation of theory development from theory application has led to a perception, by some therapists, that theory and practice are distinct entities: pre-existing theories can be learned from books and then applied to practice situations. The technical-rational approach to occupational therapy employs frames of reference and models to identify and solve the problems presented by clients. The technologist is a practitioner who works in this way: a person skilled in the application of science (*Shorter Oxford English Dictionary*, 2002).

The science of occupational therapy 'is a synthesis of knowledge adopted from many different disciplines together with concepts and theories developed within the profession and the experience of individual practitioners' (Creek, 2003, p. 32). The Swedish philosopher, Törnebohm (1991), suggested that occupational therapists require four types of knowledge:

- Knowledge in a wide sense about the world, about nature, society, culture and people;
- A view of, and ideals about, occupational therapy;
- Practical knowledge of how to work with clients;
- Interest in the people we work with and in occupational therapy.

The therapist draws on these four areas of knowledge to build an understanding of the client's life-world and to decide on the best way of working with the client.

The knowledge base of occupational therapy has expanded rapidly since the 1950s and now encompasses concepts, descriptive or explanatory models and applied theories. Occupational therapy students are exposed to theory during pre-registration education, including theories developed within occupational therapy, biomedicine, sociology, psychology and ergonomics. Most practitioners are exposed to new ideas and theories throughout their working lives, especially during times of rapid scientific discovery and change.

In order to be able to use theory effectively, the therapist has to be able to integrate explicit knowledge with practice. This involves: being able to identify dysfunction and function; understanding how people move between these two states; being able to predict how occupational therapy can influence that movement; recognising when interventions are not working, and finding more effective ways of intervening. The success of an intervention depends not only on the breadth and depth of the therapist's knowledge but also on the quality of her understanding.

A good technologist usually specialises in a particular field, learns and keeps up to date with theory and practice in that area and even, perhaps, engages in research or theory development. Some technologists take further academic courses, either in occupational therapy or in other disciplines such as psychology or sociology. The technologist defines her practice by the theories that she uses, for example, 'I use a cognitive-behavioural approach' or 'My work is based on the Canadian model of occupational performance.'

Skilled occupational therapy intervention is grounded in technical excellence and a sound understanding of the uses of theory, but not all expert occupational therapists are technicians or technologists. The American anthropologist, Cheryl Mattingly, wrote that the application of theory is a necessary condition for effective practice but is not sufficient in itself: 'One cannot do without such a grounding, but it, alone, will not yield good clinical interventions; because theoretical reasoning differs from clinical reasoning' (Mattingly, 1991, p. 980).

Mattingly went on to explain that theories are concerned with what can be reliably predicted to hold true across the majority of cases. However, the occupational therapist is not just concerned with impairment, or with discrete problems of function, but with how a health condition impacts on all aspects of a person's life, with the client's illness experience. Some practitioners accept that the outcomes of working with people in the context of their daily lives can never be entirely predictable: these therapists are able to draw on a range of theories and a store of experiential knowledge in order to find a way through complex situations. The practitioner who takes her practical skills and knowledge for granted and puts clinical reasoning in the foreground is *the thinker.*

The thinker

A thinker is 'a person who has highly developed powers of thought' (*Shorter Oxford English Dictionary*, 2002). Thinking means using the mind, exercising it in a positive, active way. It includes such mental actions as applying rules, choosing, conceptualising, evaluating, judging, justifying, knowing, perceiving and understanding. These are not exclusively professional actions but are the types of thinking used by all people as they go about their daily lives.

Thinking skills and strategies enable people to survive and to meet their needs within an increasingly complex and constantly changing world. Modern society is described as being characterised by 'uncertainty, complexity, ambivalence and disorder, a growing distrust of social institutions and traditional authorities and an increasing awareness of the threats inherent in everyday life' (Lupton, 1999, pp. 11–12). In complex, threatening situations, people have to try to understand what is going on and work out the best ways of coping, rather than responding instinctively or habitually to circumstances: thinking has become a necessary skill for human survival.

The practice of occupational therapy is not independent of its social context but is subject to the same pressures and predicaments that abound in daily life. Schön (1983, p. 14) claimed that 'complexity, uncertainty, instability, uniqueness, and value conflicts . . . are increasingly perceived as central to the world of professional practice'. This means that thinking has to be an integral part of being a professional: professional practice is not just about doing things but is about doing things thoughtfully (Nixon and Creek, 2006).

The occupational therapist has to be able to process a range of information if she is to select the most appropriate course of action with an individual client, within a specific treatment context, in order to achieve the best possible outcome. She has to be aware of, and take account of (Creek, 2003):

- Her own capabilities and limitations. For example, the therapist's age and gender will influence how her clients react to her and what she can expect to do with them.

- The elements that the client brings to the therapeutic encounter. These include his personal history and life experience, his language and culture, his thoughts, beliefs, values and aspirations, his relationships and occupations, and his needs, problems and goals.

- A multiplicity of contextual factors, such as the social environment, the setting where the therapist and client are meeting and the policy context.

In order to deal with all this information, and to incorporate it into the decision-making process, the therapist has to be able to think quickly and flexibly, using a variety of styles of thinking.

A study of how occupational therapists think in practice, commissioned in the 1980s by the American Occupational Therapy Association and the American Occupational Therapy Foundation (Mattingly and Gillette, 1991), introduced the idea of the therapist with a three-track mind. The tracks are three distinctly different ways of thinking in practice, depending on the nature of the problem being addressed and the purpose of reasoning. They are:

- **Procedural reasoning**: This is used when thinking about the disease or disability and deciding which activity to use in order to remediate the client's functional performance problems. The experienced therapist generates and tests alternative hypotheses, actively seeking and interpreting patterns of cues in order to select the most appropriate treatment medium. However, the less experienced therapist is more likely to seek what she perceives as the right answer, rather than considering multiple possibilities.

- **Interactive reasoning**: This is used during face-to-face encounters, when the therapist is trying to understand the client as an individual – what he sees as his problems, how he feels about treatment, what his likes and dislikes are and what his aspirations are. The aim is to understand the experience of illness or disability from the client's point of view – the illness perspective. This allows the therapist to match treatment aims and strategies accurately to the individual and to adjust them as the intervention progresses.

- **Conditional reasoning**: This form of reasoning places the client within his wider context. The therapist thinks about the whole experience of the client and his family, before and after the illness or accident, the social and physical contexts in which they live and the meanings that the illness or disability has for them. She thinks about alternative outcomes and possible ways in which the illness experience might change or be changed. Most importantly, the therapist involves the client fully in the construction of possible outcomes. This type of reasoning is called conditional because 'a change in the [patient's] present condition was conditional on the therapist's and the patient's participation in effective therapy. This condition was dependent . . . on building a shared image of the person's future self' (Fleming, 1991, p. 1012).

Subsequent work by Sinclair (see Chapter 8) explored further the complex and multilayered nature of thinking in occupational therapy. The Sinclair Matrix of Clinical Reasoning incorporates five distinct types of reasoning:

- **Evidence discovery** includes problem sensing, problem formulation and problem definition.
- **Theory application** is theorising in practice. This is a process of thinking about what we are doing, in collaboration with others, so that we reach a shared understanding of goals and means (Nixon and Creek, 2006).
- **Decision making** includes the three types of reasoning described by Mattingly and Fleming as they are used to evaluate, plan, set priorities, predict and determine the best treatment approach.
- **Judgement** includes reflection on practice leading to recognition of divergent views and of one's own biases.
- **Ethics** includes recognition of ethical issues, sensitivity to different views, and honesty in facing personal biases.

Mattingly and Fleming (1994), in the American clinical reasoning study, found that the way the therapist uses each type of thinking is different depending on her experience. However, the experienced therapist is able to move rapidly and smoothly from one form of thinking to another:

Reasoning styles changed as the therapist's attention was drawn from the clinical condition to another feature of the problem, and to how the person feels about the problem. Therapists could process or analyze different aspects of the problem almost simultaneously, using different thinking styles; and they did not 'lose track of' their thoughts about aspects of a problem as those components were temporarily shifted to the background while another aspect was brought into the foreground.

(Fleming, 1994, pp. 120–121)

The thinking therapist finds it difficult to say what she does, or to define her role, because practice is person-centred, that is, the intervention is directed by the client's needs and goals. The therapist does not know what techniques or theories she will use until the intervention is negotiated with the client and relevant others. She does not see herself as an expert in the client's life but recognises that the client is the expert in his own life.

The therapist who practises in a person-centred way is working in partnership with the client. Her role and approach are not predetermined but are negotiated with the client as part of the process of therapy. This means that the therapist has to pay close attention to what the client is saying, without trying to fit him into a theoretical framework that might have more to do with her own needs than with the reality of his life (Smith, 2006). In the person-centred approach, theories are tools that can be used or discarded, depending on how useful they are to the client, rather than being seen as frameworks that structure practice.

In person-centred practice, instead of relying on pre-existing theories to guide practice, the therapist uses 'a range of mental strategies and high level cognitive processes . . . to reach a decision about the best course of action' (Creek, 2003, p. 39). Decision making, in the therapeutic context, is 'a deliberative process whereby we move backwards and forwards between consideration of ends and means in order to decide upon the best possible course of action' (Nixon and Creek, 2006, p. 78). Crucially, this deliberation is done in partnership with the client: thinking can be seen as an ongoing dialogue between the therapist and client.

The technician, the technologist and the thinker are names given to three facets of the occupational therapy practitioner. They indicate approaches to different types of problem encountered within the practice of occupational therapy but they do not denote a level of skill or expertise. The expert practitioner may be highly skilled in using practical techniques, in applying theory, in thinking or in all three. In the next section, the nature of expert practice is explored.

The development of expertise

In the 1970s, the United Stated Air Force commissioned research into how pilots learn their complex, high-level skills. A mathematician and a philosopher, Dreyfus and Dreyfus (1980, in Benner, 1982), studied how chess players and pilots learn their skills and produced the Dreyfus model of skill acquisition, which describes five levels of proficiency through which the learner passes during the learning process:

1. **Novice**: The novice, or beginner, has little or no experience with the situations in which he has to work, therefore he depends on what he has been taught to guide his actions. The novice is not able to use his discretion in making judgements but has to follow context-free rules. An example of this kind of rule is a guideline taken from an American occupational therapy textbook:

> An effective way to gather information about a client's problem is to ask open-ended questions. Open-ended questions are structured so that one cannot answer them with a simple yes or no. In contrast, closed questions are so structured that one can answer only yes or no. Open-ended questions result in answers that are richer than yes or no.
>
> (Lewin and Reed, 1998, p. 52)

The novice practitioner who has learned this rule will follow it with all clients in all situations without taking account of individual differences.

2. **Advanced beginner**: After some experience, the practitioner has been in enough real practice situations to recognise salient aspects, or patterns, and can demonstrate marginally acceptable performance. The American nurse theorist, Benner (1986, p. 404), said that 'while aspects may be made explicit, they cannot be made completely objective . . . Aspect recognition is dependent on prior experience.' This means that learning to recognise patterns is an important part of the learning process for beginners and advanced beginners.

3. **Competent**: Competency typically develops when the practitioner begins to see his actions in terms of long-term goals. These goals determine which aspects of the situation are considered most important and which can be ignored. The competent practitioner is organised and efficient and has a sense of being able to cope. Most health and social care institutions expect their staff to abide by rules, protocols and standardised procedures, so the competent practitioner works comfortably within these settings.

4. **Proficient**: The proficient practitioner perceives situations as wholes rather than aspects or patterns. The current situation is compared with a range of similar experiences that the practitioner has had, so that anything unusual is immediately noticed and dealt with. Proficient performers are able to respond flexibly to changes in the situation.

5. **Expert**: At this level the practitioner no longer relies on rules or guidelines but is able to draw on a broad range of experience to sum up the situation intuitively and focus on the problem. It is difficult to describe expert practice in words because it depends on embodied knowledge that allows the practitioner to respond to changes in the environment without conscious thought. This kind of knowledge can only be gained from practical experience. Mattingly (1991, p. 979), wrote that 'Words always fall short of practice' and that 'The gap between what we can say and what we know may . . . grow as we gain professional expertise.'

Expertise in a complex skill can only be learned in practice and developed with experience. The British occupational therapist, Jenkins, in her study of how occupational therapists learn in practice, emphasised the importance of having time to learn alongside more experienced professionals (Jenkins and Brotherton, 1995). She described occupational therapy as being located within a community of practice. The essence of community is communication and interaction: 'interaction with fellow practitioners in the job, on the job and about the job [extending to] communicating with external agencies' (Jenkins and Brotherton, 1995, p. 283).

The learner, or novice therapist, starts out by being peripherally involved in the community, watching and listening to more experienced practitioners in action. Through such peripheral participation (Lave and Wenger, 1989, in Jenkins and Brotherton, 1995), the novice learns what happens in context and begins to make sense of what she sees and hears. Crucially, she learns not only how to do the job but how to do it in context. The end point of such learning is full participation in the community of practice.

The student

Occupational therapy students are novice practitioners, in the language of the Dreyfus and Dreyfus study (1980, in Benner, 1982). At the beginning of their educational programme, they have little or no experience of practice and depend on what they are taught at university to guide their actions while on practice placements.

Mastery of some basic technical skills is necessary for the student to be able to move from observing practice to trying out techniques, under supervision, in the treatment context. The student occupational therapist embarking on a first practice placement is expected to learn by observing what goes on. By the time of the next practice placement, she needs to know how to carry out core professional tasks within that setting so that she can take the first steps towards becoming a practitioner. By gaining experience in a range of practice settings, the student learns core skills and techniques for different areas of occupational therapy practice. These include transferable skills, such as communication, activity analysis and functional assessment, and specific skills for working with various health conditions.

The student also starts to learn how to apply theory in practice by observing her supervisor on the first practice placement and asking for explanations of why things are done in the way they are. By the second placement, she should be able to follow rules and guidelines that she has been taught at university, learned from books or picked up from her observations on the first placement.

Sinclair (Chapter 8) identified the thinking skills of the novice occupational therapy practitioner as limited. The student does not know what information to seek when meeting a client for the first time, and she is not able to identify which aspects of the situation to ignore and which to pay attention to. She is unable to modify what she has learned in the academic setting to suit the context of the fieldwork placement, so her application of theory is inflexible. She is slow to formulate problems and to decide what to do, and she has difficulty dealing with unfamiliar situations.

Throughout two, three or four years of study and practice placement experience, the student occupational therapist develops her practical skills, theory base and thinking skills. At the time of graduation, the new practitioner should, at the least, have reached the level of advanced beginner.

The new practitioner

The newly qualified occupational therapist, in order to be judged fit to practise, must be competent in a number of practical skills that are specified by professional bodies, such as the World Federation of Occupational Therapists (2002), and regulatory bodies, such as the Health Professions Council (2003). She must, for example, be able to: use activity analysis and synthesis to realise the therapeutic potential of occupation; adapt and apply the occupational therapy process in collaboration with individuals or populations, and work towards making environments accessible and adaptable (European Network of Occupational Therapists in Higher Education, n.d.).

The beginning therapist is expected to have a range of knowledge that can be used to guide practice until she has enough experience to pick out the salient features of a situation and make decisions about what is important in these circumstances. For example, the new graduate is expected to 'know how professional principles are expressed and translated into action through a number of different assessment, treatment and management approaches and how to select or modify approaches to meet the needs of an individual' (Health Professions Council, 2003, p. 15).

Sinclair (Chapter 8) described how the beginner is able to incorporate some contextual information into her rule-based thinking, because she has had a range of practice experience during placements. She still follows procedures but is able to recognise some patterns. However, she cannot recognise what features of a situation are important or determine priorities for action. Her practice is still slow and awkward.

As described above, some therapists choose to develop one aspect of their practice to a level of expertise while they remain merely competent in other aspects. The expert technician advances and maintains expertise in practical skills; the expert technologist understands and keeps up to date with the use of theory to direct practice; the expert thinker develops her ability to think flexibly and fluently about the situations she encounters, using different types of thinking to deal with different types of problem. But the expert occupational therapist must have expertise in all three approaches because practical skills, theory and thinking are all essential elements of effective occupational therapy practice.

The expert occupational therapist

Skilled observers of occupational therapy have described the complex, dynamic nature of occupational therapy practice and stressed the range of knowledge and skills that are required for practitioners to fulfil their demanding professional role.

In the 1970s, a sociologist, Alaszewski, undertook a comparative study of three health care professions. He observed that some professions are 'technique-oriented', in that they define their area of practice and competence in terms of a technique: for example, radiography is concerned only with patients who require that technique (Alaszewski, 1979, p. 432). In contrast, occupational therapy is 'patient-oriented', in that it is concerned with 'the social effects of disease' and with intervening 'in the social and physical environment to adjust it to the individual' (p. 432). This orientation means that occupational therapy is not limited in its application but can be of benefit to 'an expanding range of client groups' (p. 437).

A physician, Engelhardt, wrote in the 1980s that occupational therapists take different roles and move between them depending on the needs of the patient. He identified occupational therapists as both technologists, applying scientific theories to address treatment problems, and custodians of meaning, 'conveying complex services of care and guidance' (Engelhardt, 1983, p. 141).

The role of technologist requires that occupational therapists have:

> a theoretical base grounded in the internal, organic, and psychic conditions of the organisms. That is, occupational therapists function as scientist-technologists, appealing to muscular skeletal status, sensory motor and nervous system function, and intrapsychic states to aid individuals to regain and maintain as much independent function as possible.
>
> (Engelhardt, 1983, p. 141)

However, to be human is to look for meaning in events, and the people who use health care services are not only seeking treatment but also need the therapist to help them explore what it means to have a health condition. They 'want *both* a scientific account [of their condition] *and* an account in terms of their functioning in everyday life' (Engelhardt, 1983, p. 141). To satisfy this need, occupational therapists have to 'offer models of therapy which take into account not only physical capacities, but the virtues of human adaptation in recreation and in physical and mental activities generally' (p. 144). Engelhardt described this as a sacerdotal role 'in which [occupational therapists] aid individuals in orienting themselves within the changing circumstances of aging, illness and disability' (p. 143).

The anthropologist, Mattingly, also observed that occupational therapists work with more than just functional problems, 'the body as machine': they also address 'problems that go far beyond the physical body, encompassing social, cultural, and psychological issues that concern the *meaning* of illness or injury to a person's life' (Mattingly, 1994, p. 37). She described occupational therapy as a 'two-body practice' that encompasses both a disease perspective, which focuses on problem identification and treatment, and an illness experience perspective, which is concerned with the ways that disease affects a person's life (p. 37). The occupational therapist has to be able to perceive and understand the client's problems and needs from both these perspectives.

Mattingly observed that an occupational therapist can 'interweave interventions that address both the disease and the illness experience into the same treatment activity', shifting between two distinct approaches with the same patient within the same session (Mattingly, 1994, p. 38). The expert therapist is able to move easily and naturally from one approach to the other, using her clinical reasoning skills to synthesise and integrate these two types of practice.

The clinical reasoning study by Mattingly and Fleming (1994) and the Dreyfus and Dreyfus study of the acquisition and development of complex skills both describe highly skilled practice that does not just focus on a discrete problem but is responsive to the environment and ambient conditions. Both put an emphasis on the thinking skills and processes of the practitioner as she applies her practical skills to the situation. Both conceptualise the expert practitioner as one who can think in a variety of ways, who is flexible in changing her thinking to suit what is being thought about and who thinks so quickly that her decisions appear to be intuitive rather than the result of cognitive processes.

Two Danish occupational therapists, Fortmeier and Thanning, developed a model of the occupational therapy process that acknowledges the complexity of practice and offers a way of understanding how the therapist manages to keep the different strands in place over time (Fortmeier and Thanning, 2002). The model describes five tracks that represent aspects of the occupational therapist's intervention:

- **The motivation track**: this is about developing and maintaining the patient's motivation for treatment and seeking his active engagement in the process. It requires the therapist to be sensitive and responsive to the patient's changing needs.

- **The communication track**: this is about the quality of the therapeutic relationship that is necessary for an intervention to succeed. It is based on mutual respect and partnership.

- **The skills and functions track**: this concerns the patient's functional problems and the resources of the therapist for dealing with them. These resources include the therapist's practical skills and clinical reasoning.

- **The activity track**: this track is about how the therapist plans programmes of intervention and selects activities that will both meet therapeutic goals and have meaning and value for the patient.

- **The combination track**: this combines the four other tracks of the occupational therapy process with the therapist's reflections on her own actions and on the context of the intervention. It is the track in which all the elements of the situation are integrated to produce a relevant, co-ordinated and effective intervention.

Throughout the intervention process, these five tracks interact as the therapist develops, with the patient, an appropriate and effective approach to addressing the complex and dynamic pattern of illness, illness experience and adaptation that is the domain of concern of occupational therapy.

Summary and conclusion

This chapter explored the nature of occupational therapy as an individualised, contextually specific and complex intervention that requires of the practitioner a wide range of skills. It considered three ways in which occupational therapy practitioners approach their work:

- the technician, who focuses on using practical skills to solve the problems faced by her clients;
- the technologist, whose interventions are guided by theories, models and frames of reference, and
- the thinker, who uses a range of thinking skills to process complex information in order to be responsive to changing needs and circumstances.

The nature of professional expertise was discussed, drawing on studies of how people develop high-level practical skills. Some consideration was given to how occupational therapists develop expertise as technicians, technologists and thinkers.

The profession of occupational therapy needs people who have good practical skills, those who understand the value of theory in explaining and guiding practice and those who can manage the complexity of working in partnership with their clients to rebuild lives that are limited by illness or disability. The therapist may become an expert in any or all of these approaches, but true expertise in occupational therapy practice can only be achieved when they are all integrated. The expert occupational therapist is a thinker, a knower and a doer.

References

Alaszewski, A. (1979) Rehabilitation, the remedial professions and social policy. *Social Science and Medicine*, **13A**, 431–43.

Alaszewski, A. and Meltzer, H. (1979) The relationship between qualified and unqualified workers in health care: the case of the remedial therapy professions. *Sociology of Health and Illness*, **1**(3), 284–305.

Azima, H. and Wittkower, E.D. (1957) A partial field survey of psychiatric occupational therapy. *American Journal of Occupational Therapy*, **11**(1), 1–7.

Benner, P. (1982) From novice to expert. *American Journal of Nursing*, **82**, 402–7.

Christiansen, C. (2006) Foreword, in *The Kawa Model: Culturally Relevant Occupational Therapy* (ed. M.K. Iwama), Churchill Livingstone Elsevier, Edinburgh.

Creek, J. (2002) The knowledge base of occupational therapy, in *Occupational Therapy and Mental Health* (ed. J. Creek), Churchill Livingstone, Edinburgh, pp. 29–49.

Creek, J. (2003) *Occupational Therapy Defined as a Complex Intervention*, College of Occupational Therapists, London.

Creek, J., Ilott, I., Cook, S. and Munday, C. (2005) Valuing occupational therapy as a complex intervention. *British Journal of Occupational Therapy*, **68**(6), 281–4.

Engelhardt, H.T. (1983) Occupational therapists as technologists and custodians of meaning, in *Health Through Occupation: Theory and Practice in Occupational Therapy* (ed. G. Kielhofner), F.A. Davis Co., Philadelphia, pp. 139–45.

European Network of Occupational Therapists in Higher Education (n.d.) *Tuning and Quality*. (www.enothe.hva.nl) 26 September 2006.

Fleming, M.H. (1991) The therapist with the three-track mind. *American Journal of Occupational Therapy*, **45**(11), 1007–14.

Fleming, M.H. (1994) The therapist with the three-track mind, in *Clinical Reasoning: Forms of Inquiry in a Therapeutic Practice* (C. Mattingly and M.H. Fleming), F.A. Davis, Philadelphia.

Fortmeier, S. and Thanning, G. (2002) *From the Patient's Point of View: An Activity Theory Approach to Occupational Therapy*, Danish Association of Occupational Therapists, Copenhagen.

Haworth, N.A. and MacDonald, E.M. (1946) *Theory of Occupational Therapy*, Balliere, Tindall & Cox, London.

Health Professions Council (2003) *Standards of Proficiency: Occupational Therapists*, HPC, London.

Health Professions Council (n.d.) www.hpc-uk.org (20 September 2006).

Jenkins, M. and Brotherton, C. (1995) In search of a theoretical framework for practice, part 1. *British Journal of Occupational Therapy*, **58**(7), 280–5.

Lewin, J.E. and Reed, C.A. (1998) *Creative Problem Solving in Occupational Therapy*, Lippincott, Philadelphia.

Lupton, D. (1999) *Risk*, Routledge, London.

Mattingly, C. (1991) What is clinical reasoning? *American Journal of Occupational Therapy*, **45**(11), 979–86.

Mattingly, C. (1994) Occupational therapy as a two-body practice: the body as machine, in *Clinical Reasoning: Forms of Inquiry in a Therapeutic Practice* (C. Mattingly and M.H. Fleming), F.A. Davis, Philadelphia, pp. 37–63.

Mattingly, C. and Fleming, M.H. (1994) *Clinical Reasoning: Forms of Inquiry in a Therapeutic Practice*, F.A. Davis, Philadelphia.

Mattingly, C. and Gillette, N. (1991) Anthropology, occupational therapy and action research. *American Journal of Occupational Therapy*, **45**(11), 972–8.

Mendez, M.A. (1986) *A Chronicle of the World Federation of Occupational Therapists: The First Thirty Years 1952–1982*, WFOT, Jerusalem.

Meyer, A. (1977) The philosophy of occupation therapy. *American Journal of Occupational Therapy*, **31**(10), 639–42. Reprinted from *Archives of Occupational Therapy* (1922) **1**, 1–10.

Nixon, J. and Creek, J. (2006) Towards a theory of practice. *British Journal of Occupational Therapy*, **69**(2), 77–80.

O'Sullivan, E.N.M. (1955) *Textbook of Occupational Therapy: With Chief Reference to Psychological Medicine*. H.K. Lewis, London.

Paterson, C.F. (2002) A short history of occupational therapy in psychiatry, in *Occupational Therapy and Mental Health* (ed. J. Creek), Churchill Livingstone, Edinburgh, pp. 3–14.

Reilly, M. (1962) Occupational therapy can be one of the great ideas of 20th century medicine. *American Journal of Occupational Therapy*, **16**(1), 1–9.

Schön, D.A. (1983) *The Reflective Practitioner: How Professionals Think in Action*, Basic Books, New York.

Shorter Oxford English Dictionary (2002), 5th edn, Oxford University Press, Oxford.

Smith, G. (2006) The Casson Memorial Lecture 2006: Telling tales – how stories and narratives co-create change. *British Journal of Occupational Therapy*, **69**(7), 304–11.

Törnebohm, H. (1991) What is worth knowing in occupational therapy? *American Journal of Occupational Therapy*, **45**(5), 451–4.

Wilcock, A. (1998) A theory of occupation and health, in *Occupational Therapy: New Perspectives* (ed. J. Creek), Whurr Publishers Ltd., London, pp. 1–15.

World Federation of Occupational Therapists (2002) *Minimum Standards for the Education of Occupational Therapists*, WFOT.

World Health Organization (2001) *ICF: International Classification of Functioning, Disability and Health*. WHO, Geneva.

The romance of occupational therapy

2

Clare Hocking

Introduction

Occupational therapists working in Britain in the 1930s longed to show doctors that their fledgling profession achieved significant health outcomes. Although they had few tools with which to measure its effectiveness, they did what they could. They recorded the number of men and women attending occupation centres and their diagnoses, and accounted for the craft materials bought and the finished items sold. Yet these statistics and careful accounts did not show what was accomplished. To achieve that, therapists recorded their observations of patients transformed by their encounter with occupational therapy.

This chapter recalls a number of those accounts, revealing them to be tales of triumph over physical, intellectual and psychiatric conditions; of skill, hope and self-respect emerging from hopelessness and despair. Underlying those stories are the profession's Romantic assumptions about the curative power of art and craftwork. A central notion was that unleashing people's creativity might help them transcend the stultifying effects of incapacity, hospitalisation and industrial labour. Where those beliefs came from and how they shaped the profession is the subject of this discussion. It also charts the complex reasons occupational therapists moved away from craftwork, and how Romantic perspectives nonetheless survived to inform the profession's philosophical assumptions.

Early accounts of effectiveness

Three early accounts, by a doctor, a medical superintendent and an occupational therapist, have been selected as examples of outcomes attributed to occupational therapy. They are drawn from different settings and different countries, yet they are representative of many stories told in the early literature. Each describes a patient or patients who were radically changed. They are presented here in the words of the original author. First, however, aspects of the medical, social and attitudinal context of these stories are outlined. This contextual information is provided because accounts of human action and motives are written in a particular place and time, and incorporate contemporary norms and expectations. To fully appreciate the meaning of a story, it is necessary to understand something of that background.

The fact that occupational therapists worked in medical and psychiatric settings is an important part of what shaped the assumptions they made and the ways they worked. Glimpses of what was happening in hospitals in Britain between the two world wars are afforded within the occupational therapy literature itself. A particular feature was the lengthy hospitalisation that many patients experienced, although improvements were being made. For example, in 1935, people with a fractured patella who were seen in a fracture clinic averaged 26 weeks off work, compared to 57 weeks for those treated elsewhere (Plewes, 1951). Such dramatic reductions in treatment time were the result of a fundamental shift in medical management. Previously, it had been thought that the best treatment for any trauma, whether a fracture or a leucotomy, was a period of complete rest (Sicely, 1950). In orthopaedic settings, the negative consequences of prolonged immobilisation were taken as a given. Dr Elizabeth Casson (1938/39), for example, cited restoration of shoulder movement after a fracture of the humerus as a standard occupational therapy intervention. In so doing, she indicates that loss of movement at the shoulder was an accepted outcome of a fracture of the upper arm. Moreover, protracted hospitalisations were a common outcome of many ailments, not just orthopaedic conditions. For instance, even in 1947 the average stay in a tuberculosis sanatorium was 500 days (Cox, 1947). Being apart from society for such lengthy periods contributed to many patients losing confidence in their ability to return to normal life, as well as losing the general fitness required to do so. In addition, it was accepted that some patients, including many in psychiatric hospitals, would never return to life outside the hospital walls.

As well as anticipating that it would take a long time to get well, people had much lower expectations of recovery. In his address to the 1951 occupational therapy conference, for example, Lord Amulree mentioned in passing that if patients were admitted following a stroke 'you may have them for a year or more, gradually improving all the time' (Amulree, 1951, p. 214). He went on to note that because people generally believed that stroke victims weren't 'much good for anything' (p. 215), therapists would need to convince patients that they could still do something. Similarly, John Colson (1945) pointed out that 'before beginning occupational therapy the patient may not be completely convinced that his injury can be cured, or that it will not prevent him from carrying out normal activities' (p. 6). In addition to expecting little from rehabilitation, patients could not look forward to much in the way of social acceptance or financial support. In the absence of unemployment or sickness benefits, men in particular faced the immediate worry of how their family was faring on a substantially reduced income, and the more distant worry of their future employability (Smith, 1945). In the United States at least, destitution was one acknowledged outcome of acquiring a disability (Hudson and Fish, 1944).

Against this background of understanding, the stories of four individuals who benefited from occupational therapy are now related. The first is by Dr Elizabeth Casson, who established the first school of occupational therapy in England. It comes from her presentation to the Conference on 'Welfare of Cripples and Invalid Children' in London in 1935.

> Not long ago Miss Forrester Brown invited one of my Occupational Therapy staff to work under her at the Bath Orthopaedic Hospital, and prescribed occupations for a man with an injured spine. Lying near him were two boys who had lately come to the Hospital from remote farms. They had had infantile paralysis when quite young. Their families had settled down to the fact that they were cripples. They had been washed and fed quite kindly, and that was all. During the long years they had become completely apathetic and seemingly feeble-minded. They lay in bed in Hospital and watched the man in the next bed. Gradually curiosity was stimulated by what they saw and heard and they began to want to do something too. One boy asked for a pencil, and when he saw his drawing and felt his muscles producing his drawing, a whole new life came to him. Both boys are now working well, and quickly showed their intelligence is excellent.
>
> (Casson, 1955, p. 99)

The second story is by Silvia Docker, who trained as an occupational therapist in England and subsequently become an important figure in the establishment of the profession in Australia. While Casson's account is couched in the matter-of-fact tones befitting her status as a doctor, Docker (1938/1939) was more emotive in her report of working with a young Australian woman.

> I had a bad Spastic case while I was in Melbourne and I tried her on chair-caning. The first day I found she was so bad that she could hardly get into the room;

her arms and legs went in all directions. I showed her how to wind the cane to soak it, but she kept breaking it. I then helped her to get the cane through the holes. She couldn't reach the further side of the chair and after half-an-hour she had only managed to get her cane through one hole from the underside. She asked if she could try when I was not there, and I said 'of course', but I made an effort to go to her two days later as I felt I had expected too much and must get her on to something else before she lost heart. To my amazement her mother brought in the chair with the first two rows of caning done. I asked how much the mother had helped and was told not at all, she had persisted on her own. . . . She was already planning about the trade she would do at chair mending. She is sixteen and the Doctors had told her mother not to bother with her that she would never walk or even learn to read.

(Docker, 1938/39, p. 28)

Similar stories of achievements that exceeded all expectations were told about patients in psychiatric hospitals. The example cited here comes from John Ivison Russell, the medical superintendent of North Riding Mental Hospital and an examiner in occupational therapy to the Association of Occupational Therapists. In his book describing *The Occupational Treatment of Mental Illness*, Russell (1938) gave the following account of successes wrought in a male occupation centre:

In one part of the room two patients are making galvanised wire netting. Both patients are epileptic, and one is further handicapped by infantile hemiplegia. Before admission to the mental hospital he was graded as a moral imbecile, profane in language and vicious in habits. He is now thoroughly proud of himself and the muscular development that has resulted from turning the wheel, and his general conduct is consistently good. His companion was for many years a quarrelsome and disagreeable man, and was classed as turbulent and unemployable, but his keen interest and pride in the manufacture of wire fencing has completely socialised him.

(Russell, 1938, pp. 92–3)

These are remarkable outcomes, brought about by simple activities: using a pencil, being shown how to weave chair seating, turning a wheel to make wire netting. Such claims reflect early occupational therapists' belief in the potency of art and craft activities. They, like the doctors who supported the profession in its early days, were fully confident that creating something would 'rouse [patients] out of their hopeless lethargy' (Thornely, 1948, p. 24). Furthermore, therapists took it for granted that illness might 'enhance, distort or release' a patient's 'hidden potentialities' (English, 1946, p. 13), and that this latent talent would emerge through making things. Accordingly, simple crafts such as fabric printing might 'open up vistas' and lead to the discovery of personal qualities 'hitherto unknown and unsuspected' (Rivett, 1938/39, p. 20). In the process, self-respect and self-reliance would be restored. Furthermore, the things patients made would stand testament to their transformation. Patients' paintings, for example, were described as intimate records of the soul's 'pain and struggle – its defeat and brokenness – its triumph and resurrection' (Champernowne, 1952, pp. 157–8). Equally, however, poorly chosen activities would bring 'disappointment and disillusionment' (McLuskie, 1940, p. 8), 'plunge the patient still further into a confused, depressed state of mind' (English, 1940, p. 18), or induce suicidal despondency (*Journal of the Occupational Therapists Association,* 1938/39). Of concern here is how occupational therapists came to believe that the work they did could have such results. That is the topic of the next section.

Romantic assumptions

What the stories told have in common is that these patients, each previously considered a hopeless case, were transformed by the simple expedient of doing some artwork or learning a craft. Two things are noteworthy in this regard. First, like William Morris who held that 'all men can learn some useful craft' (1886/1936, p. 489), the early occupational therapists seem never to have doubted that all patients had a natural talent for one craft or another. The therapist's skill lay in selecting the right one (Baily, 1938). Second, no explanation of how the change came about seems necessary and none is offered, save that the person engaged in a craft. There is no sense of hard-won behavioural change over an extended period, although that might have been the case. There is no talk of graded skill development through increasingly complex activities, or teaching less demanding steps of the task first. Rather, Docker teaches chair caning in its logical sequence, starting with soaking the cane to make it supple and threading it through the holes. Neither is there any hint of contemporary concerns such as client choice or the personal meaningfulness of the task, although consistent with the established wisdom of the times the tasks were likely chosen with the patient's gender in mind. What is presented is that patients learned an art technique or craft and as a result they were radically changed. True to the spirit of Romanticism, such claims are presented in the manner of magnificent and self-evident truths.

Another feature of these stories is the sense of excitement and triumph that emerges from them. Whether couched in Casson's constrained medical style, or Docker's unguarded anxiety over giving too demanding a task and astonishment that the girl succeeded, an intensity of emotion is evident. This emotionality is reminiscent of the Romantics, who valued creativity, self-expression and fully living one's emotions (Saiedi, 1993; Tarnas, 1996). They also believed that everyone has the potential to transcend their circumstances and discover their spiritual essence, and that this was best achieved through extreme experiences (Pioch, 1995). Given the prevailing attitudes towards disability, such that families discarded their sons as 'cripples', mothers were advised not bother with their daughters, and patients could be characterised as unemployable imbeciles, having a mental illness or physical disability might well be considered an extreme experience. Russell (1938), for example, described mental illness in terms of a 'troubled mind . . . seeking refuge in morbid introspection in which it can find but a nightmare of unworthiness and despair' (p. 8). Similarly, Docker (1938/1939) referred in passing to 'the inferiority complex that all people with physical disability must get' (p. 29). In the context of such attitudes, even among health professionals, being recognised as intelligent, committed to learning a trade, or keenly interested is indeed a triumph.

Also noteworthy in the stories that were told is the nature of the transformation reported. The storytellers don't concentrate on improved co-ordination, greater strength or enhanced social skills. Their language points to change in the patients themselves, and to emotionally charged outcomes. A whole new life came into them. They were thoroughly proud of their accomplishments. Docker's spastic case for the first time envisioned a future in which she might have a place as a worker. Yet despite the pleasure evident in the telling, these stories are recorded as completely within the realms of what occupational therapy might be expected to achieve. Such stories bear all the hallmarks of Romanticism, which envisions creative genius arising from chaos and asserts the human potential to transcend the drudgery of daily life and be heroically transformed (Saiedi, 1993). In the stories told of patients' triumphs, it is not day-to-day drudgery that is transcended but the terrible adversity of disease and handicap.

Occupational therapy's roots in Romanticism

How, then, did occupational therapists come to believe that getting patients to paint or draw, or teaching them a craft, might bring about such revelatory change? The answer lies, largely, in the profession's link with the Arts and Crafts Movement, which flourished over the relatively short period between 1875 and 1920. Arising from widespread denouncement of the hardships endured by many factory workers, the Arts and Crafts Movement brought together a Romantic belief in the transformative power of 'noble labour' with abhorrence for shoddy, mass-produced products and industrial work. In its place, proponents imagined a return to the dignity of old-fashioned craftsmanship, brought about by a revival of the traditional arts and crafts familiar to many occupational therapists: bookbinding, weaving, canework and woodwork, basketry, metal work, pottery and so on.

Two leading proponents of the Movement, John Ruskin (1819–1900) and William Morris (1834–96), are particularly associated with occupational therapy, one in person and the other through his writings. Ruskin was an English art and social critic who railed against the neo-classical architecture of his day. He held the opinion that forcing tradesmen to be 'servile' to the pre-established rules and forms of neo-classical conventions quashed any possibility of expressing themselves through their work. In contrast he argued that Gothic architecture, with all its inherent irregularities and imperfections, gave men the freedom to represent the divine glory of the natural world in their own way (Spretnak, 1997). True to his Romantic beliefs, Ruskin asserted that being given licence to express themselves allowed craftsmen to fully become what they could be. Crafting beautiful objects by hand would enhance their spirituality and creativity, making them emotionally expressive and self-determining. In contrast, tending machines forced labourers to repeat a single action on identical components, which demeaned them and rendered them machine-like. In a particularly virulent attack, Ruskin argued that:

We have much studied and much perfected, of late, the great civilized invention of the division of labour; only we give it a false name. It is not, truly speaking, the labour that is divided; but the men: – Divided into mere segments of men – broken into small fragments and crumbs of life; so that all the little piece of intelligence that is left in a man is not enough to make a pin, or a nail, but exhausts itself in making the point of a pin or the head of a nail. Now it is a good and desirable thing, truly, to make many pins in a day; but if we could only see with what crystal sand their points were polished, – sand of human soul, much to be magnified before it can be discerned for what it is – we should think there might be some loss in it also.

(Ruskin, 1853/1964, p. 283)

In place of factory production lines, Ruskin proposed a massive reorganisation of work processes, whereby each item would be individually crafted and adorned by hand. The value of such an object, he proposed, would lie in 'discovering in it the record of thoughts, and intents, and trials, and heartbreakings – of recoveries and joyfulnesses of success' (Ruskin, 1849, p. 235). The maker of such an object, in Ruskin's view, would experience the dignity and pleasure of labour, the honour of achieving something difficult, and the identity of a handicraftsman, someone who expresses his emotions and himself in all he creates. Clearly, occupational therapists working in England in the early years of the profession ascribed to the same philosophies: that people project themselves into the things they create and that there is pleasure and honour in making things.

As Wilcock (2002) discovered, there is a direct connection between Ruskin and key individuals in occupational therapy's history in Britain. The link runs via Octavia Hill, who was a business associate and friend of Ruskin's for many years. Hill was a remarkable woman who established a programme of rehabilitating slum tenements in London. From Hill, Ruskin's philosophies passed to Elizabeth Casson who was at that time one of Hill's estate managers and also managed an activity programme for some of her tenants.

Casson's exposure to the philosophies of the Arts and Crafts Movement was furthered in the mid-1920s, after she graduated as a doctor. On a visit to the United States, she spent time in both an occupational therapy department in New York and the Boston School of Occupational Therapy. The emergent profession Casson discovered in America was itself informed by Arts and Crafts ideals. George Edward Barton, one of the founders of the National Society for the Promotion of Occupational Therapy, was the first secretary of the Boston Society of Arts and Crafts (Peloquin, 1991). Similarly Jane Addams, another important figure in the profession's beginnings, was inspired by Ruskin's *Unto This Last*, which describes the perils of industrialisation. She was subsequently involved in the establishment of the Chicago Arts and Crafts Society (Breines, 1990). Motivated by what she had seen in the States, Casson returned to England and organised occupational therapy treatment in the sanatorium at which she worked. Soon after, she founded the first School of Occupational Therapy in the United Kingdom (Wilcock, 2002).

As indicated earlier, the pioneering occupational therapists were also inspired by William Morris, but his influence seems to have been played out through his writings rather than in person. Morris was an English designer, craftsman, poet and socialist. Following in Ruskin's footsteps, Morris also became a leading figure in the Arts and Crafts Movement and, like Ruskin, he was a Romantic (Kinna, 2000). In his many public lectures and voluminous writings, Morris translated Romantic philosophies into an Arts and Crafts ideal. In particular he turned the possibility of discovering one's spiritual essence, by fully living one's emotions and unleashing human potential through creativity, into a vision of pouring one's soul into making beautiful, utilitarian objects. In crafting an object, Morris believed, the craftsman would craft himself.

Traces of Morris's ideas are readily apparent in the early occupational therapy literature. For example, his assertion that 'pleasure and interest in the work itself are necessary to the production of a work of art however humble' (Morris, 1901, p. 14) is echoed in advice given to therapists that their success hinged on stimulating interest and inducing a 'pleasant mental attitude' in the patient (Dunton, 1945, p. 5). Accordingly, therapists were instructed to 'find work that absorbs their whole attention' (Haworth and Macdonald, 1944, p. 20). Creating well-made, useful and attractive things, they were told, would 'draw on the ingenuity and gifts of self, and provide outlets for the personality' (Cooper, 1940, p. 5). However simple the product, if patients were to be given responsibility 'for the form and character' of their work, they would have an 'opportunity for self expression' (Challoner, 1948, p. 21). If occupational therapists could achieve all that, despite limitations of staff and time, they would fulfil their responsibility to regenerate patients' spirits. Work that did not 'prove congenial and make a personal appeal to the patient', however, would nullify the therapeutic effect and result in 'fatigue and ennui' (O'Sullivan, 1955, p. 23).

Induction into an Arts and Crafts mentality seems to have been implicit in the original occupational therapy training although in Britain, as in the United States, it likely came from the craftsmen employed to teach students practical skills rather than being formally taught (Breines, 1990; Serrett, 1985). Arts and Crafts perspectives are evident, for example, in Faith Johnson's (1947) report of her impressions of occupational therapy training in Britain when she visited in the mid-1940s. For instance, she noted the 'high degree of craftsmanship achieved particularly in such training schools as St. Loyes' (Johnson, 1947, p. 16). Similarly, Dunton (1945) declared good craftsmanship to be an essential qualification of American occupational therapists. References to craftsmanship and creativity are frequent, and the ideal of creating objects of both utility and beauty was regularly repeated. In 1951, the key tenets of the Arts and Crafts movement, along with its anathema of mass production, were exhorted at some length:

> *Craftsmanship* is that combination of a love of beauty with utilitarianism . . . The efficiency and economy of machine-made articles has threatened to entirely stifle the . . . human desire to make with our own hands the things needed for household and personal use and adornment, and if we are wise we will teach . . . ourselves the value and superiority of hand-made things. We will not neglect this wholesome and useful form of aesthetic self-expression.
>
> This projection of the self, especially the emotional self, into objective and permanent forms is highly valuable as a means of materialising the life of the imagination. It is essentially an expression of feeling . . .
>
> The love of *Beauty* is in itself probably the highest form of aspiration of which the human soul is capable.
>
> (Severn, 1951, pp. 115–16)

In this passage, several ideas promoted by Ruskin and Morris are synthesised: the union of beauty and utility in handcrafted objects, that the things people make express something of themselves, and the soulfulness of true craftsmanship. Morris's assumptions about the engagement of the human spirit in the act of crafting an object are perhaps best illustrated in this extract from his 1885 essay *Useful Work Versus Useless Toil*:

. . . a man at work, making something which he feels will exist because he is working at it and wills it, is exercising the energies of his mind and soul as well as his body. Memory and imagination help him as he works. Not only his own thoughts, but the thoughts of the men of past ages guide his hands; and, as a part of the human race, he creates.

(Morris, 1885/1915, p. 100)

The implicit relationship Morris perceived between the work of the hands and people's mind and will is clearly echoed in Mary Reilly's declaration that 'man through the use of his hands as they are energized by mind and will, can influence the state of his own health' (Reilly, 1962, p. 2). By the time Reilly penned this mantra for the profession, however, occupational therapy's original vision of engaging clients in crafting things had almost slipped out of everyday practice.

The decline of craftwork in occupational therapy

Although both Romantic and Arts and Crafts philosophies are clearly evident in the early occupational therapy literature, the heroic stories therapists told gradually disappeared over time. A range of complex professional and historical factors conspired to bring this about. Perhaps foremost was the profession's move away from using craft as its primary therapeutic medium. One contributing factor was that during the Second World War many occupational therapists were redeployed from mental hospitals to treat the war wounded. Instead of crafts, they set their patients to work assembling things required for the war effort. The general enthusiasm for industrial tasks extended as far as geriatric daycare settings (Wilcock, 2002).

Although the move away from crafts was contested at the time, occupational therapists' new focus on workplace skills was reinforced by a government-level focus on vocational rehabilitation. By the war's end, the Association forthrightly asserted that 'Occupational Therapists must be prepared to relegate the arts and crafts to their proper place' (*Journal of the Association of Occupational Therapists*, 1946, p. 11), which was not, apparently, in preparing patients to return to the competitive world of work. In the general enthusiasm to rebuild the nation, even people with disabilities were viewed as potential workers. In this context, arguments about the importance of developing satisfying leisure pursuits (Challoner, 1948) or crafts being a vital alternative to the strenuous recreations enjoyed by healthy people (Jones, 1947) were not sufficiently persuasive. Crafts might assist in restoring people to 'the fullest productivity' (*Occupational Therapy*, 1950, pp.

3–4) and protect and enhance health, but they were increasingly positioned as hobbies rather than the mainstay of intervention. Perhaps particularly influential in this regard was a report detailing the training requirements, job openings, likely remuneration and long working hours of craftsmen at that time. Undertaken by a group of occupational therapists, it amply demonstrated the very limited potential of the crafts they taught to lead to open employment (Jackson *et al.*, 1956). Soon, occupational therapists were talking about creating 'a "normal" workaday atmosphere' in their departments (*Occupational Therapy*, 1957a, p. 36). To ready injured industrial workers for 'the impact shock of hammers on metal' (*Occupational Therapy*, 1957b, p. 21), and rebuild their confidence to operate lathes and train as welders, some introduced industrial machinery into occupational therapy workshops.

At much the same time, occupational therapists were introduced to 'gadgets' to assist people to complete self-care and domestic tasks independently. This opportunity to shake the profession free of its disparaging image as 'arts and crafts ladies' was rapidly taken up by therapists in Britain, Australia, New Zealand, the United States and other western countries (Hocking and Wilcock, 1997). Domestic rehabilitation, with its emphasis on accomplishing daily living activities, flourished. Medical advances also had their impact. As previously mentioned, hospitalisations were becoming shorter. This challenged both the ways occupational therapists used crafts, and the need to do so. Interventions to restore self-confidence or mobilise patients after extended bed rest, for example, became less relevant. As one physician proclaimed, orthopaedic 'patients will never produce a nice-looking handbag or a rug for the bedside – they won't be with you long enough!' (Plewes, 1951, p. 65). Another innovation, the advent of teamwork, also seems to have taken its toll on craftwork as a staple of the profession. Although not commented on in the early literature, as occupational therapists increasingly subscribed to the teamwork model, they appear to have adopted the biomechanical, psychodynamic and neurodevelopmental theories promoted by other team members. Accordingly, they put aside Romantic explanations of the transformations achieved by craftwork and talked instead of attending to psychological needs, suppressed aggression, catharsis, patterns of co-ordination and reflex-inhibiting postures.

Romanticism in contemporary practice

As this discussion has shown, occupational therapy's roots in Romanticism were embedded in its adoption of arts and crafts as the primary means of intervention. As crafts were displaced over time, however, so too were claims of transforming patients. In their place, rational explanations of measured change were given, informed by a wide range of theoretical constructs. Nonetheless, Romantic notions have survived, albeit largely unrecognised. Five ideas that have endured over time are discussed to support this claim.

The first is the longstanding controversy over whether the product or process of therapy is more important. Although less evident in the current literature, determining whether the focus should be on achieving a high-quality product, something patients can be proud of, or the process of making it has been argued from the earliest literature till well into the 1980s. On one hand, if the curative factor is the experience of skilfully applying oneself to a creative act, then the craftsmanship the patient develops is more important and feedback should focus on perfecting those skills. Alternately, if exercising one's capacities to regain function of body or mind is paramount, then *how* the patient works is more significant than the skill developed. In this case, the focus should be on what the occupation requires of patients and what they actually do, and poor-quality products should be accepted or even applauded. The lack of resolution of this debate has resulted, at times, in some rather bizarre practices. Stow (1958), for instance, reported 'a tendency for occupational therapists and technicians' who 'like to see a job well done, and strive too much for absolute perfection' (p. 87) making the product for the patient rather than see it badly finished. Although such practices might readily be dismissed as an archaic curiosity, this practice survived into the 1980s when I observed occupational therapy aides unpicking and reworking the basketry efforts of elderly patients attending a creative workshop.

Alongside this debate, creativity has been an enduring topic in the profession's discourse. For example, Bing's account of the evolution of the profession suggests 'craft is a way in which man may create and cross a bridge within himself and center himself in his own essential unity' (Bing, 1981, p. 515). Repeating a familiar refrain of the Arts and Crafts Movement, Bing continued, 'his material modifies him as he modifies it'. Other references are more oblique, merely noting occupational therapy's early assumption that people are by nature 'productive, aesthetic, playful, creative, and reflective' (Kielhofner and Burke, 1977, p. 681). Still others cite creativity but link its place in the profession to recent sources (Hasselkus and Rosa, 1997). Creativity is cited as an indicator of the therapeutic value of an occupation or as contributing to well-being (Yerxa, 1998). Children's play has been has been assumed to develop the repertoire of cognitive and behavioural skills needed for creative endeavours later in life (Parham and Fazio, 1997). In addition, creative occupations have recently been identified as having the potential to invoke people's spirit (Rose, 1999) or to provide opportunities to express one's spirit (McColl, 2000). Being creative has also been associated with experiencing flow, Csikszentmihalyi's term for transcending awareness of self, place and time (Collins, 1998; do Rozario, 1994;

Toomey, 1999). Moreover, Howard and Howard (1997), echoing earlier assumptions, reached the conclusion that disability 'separates us from our active, creative, reflective potential' (p. 183). Despite the fact that such references have been ongoing, however, the profession's assumptions about creativity have not been substantively researched. Accordingly, understanding of the nature of creativity and the transformative process it might elicit has not progressed, although the occupational science symposium on creativity convened in Britain in 2004 and Schmid's (2005) scholarly exploration of creativity may signal a turning of the tide.

A third enduring notion that has its roots in the profession's Romantic past is the art of practice. Generally incorporated in the phrase 'the art and science of practice', art here refers to those aspects of being an occupational therapist not explainable in rational terms. It is the art of establishing a therapeutic alliance with a client, the art of the 'just right' challenge, the art of uncovering precisely which occupations lie at the heart of a client's identity and make his or her life worth living. Implicit in most discussions of the art of practice is the idea that it must be learned through experience, not taught, and that this is the source of occupational therapy's power to effect change.

The two final ideas of note in this discussion are holism and spirituality. Like the art of practice, these concepts suggest that there is more to practice than just science. The essence of holism is that 'the whole is more than the sum of the parts' and the concept of holistic treatment has been termed a foundational premise of the profession (Hemphill-Pearson and Hunter, 1997). In a practice context, holism suggests that facts and figures can never sum up a client, that our 'feel' for who that person is, what he or she needs and how he or she might respond, will always exceed the data generated by structured assessments or observations of task performance. Likewise, spirituality reaches beyond objective facts about physical or mental capacities; productive, self-care and leisure occupations; physical, social or institutional environments (Townsend, 2002). Yet, spirit enlivens and is revealed through all of these. The emerging discourse of spirituality points to the importance of relating to each client as a unique being, to being empathetic and hopeful, and to always remembering that we cannot predict what might be important to individuals and what might touch them (Belcham, 2004; Collins, 1998; Howard and Howard, 1997; Spencer et al., 1997). The concept of spirituality is emerging as central to discussions of client-centred practice, reminding us to strive to understand what is meaningful to people, and to never underestimate their strength, capacity and potential for achievement despite circumstances that might threaten to overwhelm them (Hammell, 2001; Unruh et al., 2002). These are Romantic notions indeed.

Conclusion

At the dawn of the profession in Britain, occupational therapy was imbued with Romantic assumptions about what might be achieved and how that might come to pass. As this discussion has shown, those understandings entered the profession, largely, through Arts and Crafts philosophies. As crafts receded from being the major tool of the profession, however, Romantic claims of the triumphs clients achieved in occupational therapy were replaced with more rational explanations. Nonetheless Romantic notions survived to inform the way occupational therapists relate to their clients and their understanding of human potential.

In losing sight of the origin of such notions, however, it seems that occupational therapists relegated their Romantic beliefs about clients to the realms of 'underground practice'. That is, they maintained a façade of rational explanations to account for what they do, why they do it, and what might be achieved while yearning for practice the way it 'should' be. This was not a longing for the crafts of old, or not necessarily. It was a sense that there should be more to practice than bath boards and shower assessments, work simplification and skills training; that there ought to be a place for acknowledging the trials and heartbreakings of disability, along with the triumph of recreating a life.

Recent developments in occupational therapy suggest that occupational therapy is rediscovering its essence as a Romantic profession. In particular, the intense focus on client-centredness and spirituality indicates a return to the implicit hopefulness of the early literature. This time around, that hopefulness is centred on the robustness of the human spirit and how it might be unlocked through occupation, that the ordinary and extraordinary things that people do might touch their spirit and transform them. This is a broader conceptualisation than the original crafts vision, but nonetheless contains its critical ingredients: engaging in things that have a personal appeal, bringing their whole attention to the task, opportunities for self-expression by controlling the form and nature of the work, and promoting ingenuity, self-reliance and self-respect.

References

Amulree, Rt. Hon. Lord (1951) Geriatrics and occupational therapy. *Occupational Therapy*, **14**(4), 213–16.

Baily, J. (1938) Cord knotting as a therapeutic measure. *Journal of the Occupational Therapists' Association*, **1**(Summer), 20–2.

Belcham, C. (2004) Spirituality in occupational therapy: theory in practice? *British Journal of Occupational Therapy*, **67**(1), 39–46.

Bing, R.K. (1981) Occupational therapy revisited: a paraphrastic journey. *American Journal of Occupational Therapy*, **35**(8), 499–518.

Breines, E. (1990) Genesis of occupation: a philosophical model for therapy and theory. *Australian Occupational Therapy Journal*, **37**(1), 45–9.

Casson, E. (1938/39) The prescription in occupational therapy. *Journal of the Occupational Therapists' Association*, **1**(Winter), 22–4.

Casson, E. (1955) Occupational therapy. *Occupational Therapy*, **18**(3), 98–100 (reprinted from Report on Conference on 'Welfare of Cripples and Invalid Children' held at the Drapers' Hall, London, on 7–8 November 1935).

Challoner, M. (1948) Is art necessary? *Journal of the Association of Occupational Therapists*, **11**(April), 20–1.

Champernowne, H.I. (1952) Art therapy. *Occupational Therapy*, **15**(4), 155–65.

Collins, M. (1998) Occupational therapy and spirituality: reflecting on quality of experience in therapeutic interactions. *British Journal of Occupational Therapy*, **61**, 280–4.

Colson, J.H.C. (1945) *The Rehabilitation of the Injured: Occupational Therapy*, Cassell & Co., London.

Cooper, V. (1940) Embroidery and the mental patient. *Journal of the Association of Occupational Therapists*, **3**(Spring), 5–7.

Cox, P.L. (1947) Occupational therapy with the tuberculous. *Journal of the Association of Occupational Therapists*, **10**(TB Supplement), 7–11.

do Rozario, L. (1994) Ritual, meaning and transcendence: the role of occupation in modern life. *Journal of Occupational Science: Australia*, **1**, 46–52.

Docker, S.B. (1938/39) Occupational therapy for orthopaedic cases. *Journal of the Occupational Therapists' Association*, **1**(Winter), 24–9.

Dunton, W.R. (1945) *Prescribing Occupational Therapy*, 2nd edn, Charles C. Thomas, Springfield, IL.

English, A.M. (1940) The use of waste materials. *Journal of the Association of Occupational Therapists*, **3**(Winter), 18–22.

English, A.M. (1946) Book review: Art versus illness. *Journal of the Association of Occupational Therapists*, **9**(No. 24), 12–14.

Hammell, K.W. (2001) Intrinsicality: reconsidering spirituality, meaning(s) and mandates. *Canadian Journal of Occupational Therapy*, **68**(3), 186–94.

Hasselkus, B.R. and Rosa, S.A. (1997) Meaning and occupation, in *Occupational Therapy: Enabling Function and Well-being*, 2nd edn (eds C. Christiansen and C. Baum), Slack, Thorofare, NJ, pp. 364–77.

Haworth, N.A. and Macdonald, M.E. (1944) *Theory of Occupational Therapy*, 2nd edn, Baillière, Tindall & Cox, London.

Hemphill-Pearson, B.J. and Hunter, M. (1997) Holism in mental health practice. *Occupational Therapy in Mental Health*, **13**(2), 35–49.

Hocking, C. and Wilcock, A. (1997) Occupational therapists as object users: a history of Australian practice 1954–1995. *Australian Occupational Therapy Journal*, **44**, 167–76.

Howard, B.S. and Howard, J.R. (1997) Occupation as spiritual activity. *American Journal of Occupational Therapy*, **51**(3), 181–5.

Hudson, H. and Fish, M. (1944) *Occupational Therapy in the Treatment of the Tuberculous Patient*, National Tuberculosis Association, New York.

Jackson, E.M., Keummel, L., Draper, S.E., Maggs, S., Thompson, G., Nott, C. and Lee, P.A. (1956) Vocational activities: report on economic possibilities and training required. *Occupational Therapy*, **19**(2), 51–6.

Jones, M.S. (1947) The connection of occupational therapy with industry. *Journal of the Association of Occupational Therapists*, **10**(January), 9–11.

Johnson, F. (1947) Some impressions of a New Zealand occupational therapist. *Journal of the Association of Occupational Therapists*, **10**(July), 16–17.

Journal of the Occupational Therapists' Association (1938/39) Address by Dr. Soltau. *Journal of the Occupational Therapists' Association*, **1**(Winter), 10–11.

Journal of the Association of Occupational Therapists (1946) The future of occupational therapy. *Journal of the Association of Occupational Therapists*, **9**(26), 10–12.

Kielhofner, G. and Burke, J.P. (1977) Occupational therapy after 60 years: an account of changing identity and knowledge. *American Journal of Occupational Therapy*, **31**(10), 675–89.

Kinna, R. (2000) *William Morris: The Art of Socialism*, University of Wales Press, Cardiff.

McColl, M.A. (2000) Spirit, occupation and disability. *Canadian Journal of Occupational Therapy*, **67**(4), 217–28.

McLuskie, D. (1940) The disposal of patients' work. *Journal of the Association of Occupational Therapists*, **3**(Spring), 7–9.

Morris, W. (1901) Art and its producers: a lecture delivered in Liverpool in 1888, in *Art and its Producers, and the Arts and Crafts of Today: Two addresses delivered before the National Association for the Advancement of Art*, Longman & Co., London, pp. 1–20.

Morris, W. (1915) Useful work versus useless toil, in *The Collected Works of William Morris. Volume XXIII. Signs of change; Lectures on socialism* (ed. M. Morris), Longman Green & Co., London, pp. 98–120 (original published 1885).

Morris, W. (1936) The reward of genius, in *William Morris: Artist, Writer, Socialist. Volume II* (ed. M. Morris), Russell & Russell, New York (original published in *The Commonweal*, 25 September 1886).

Occupational Therapy (1950) Editorial. *Occupational Therapy*, **13**(2), 3–4.

Occupational Therapy (1957a) Power tools in occupational therapy. *Occupational Therapy*, **20**(3), 36.

Occupational Therapy (1957b) Occupational therapy at Condreville. *Occupational Therapy*, **20**(2), 21–2.

O'Sullivan, E.N.M. (1955) *Textbook of Occupational Therapy: With Chief Reference to Psychological Medicine*, H.K. Lewis, London.

Parham, D. and Fazio, L.S. (eds) (1997) *Play in Occupational Therapy for Children*. Mosby, St Louis, MO.

Peloquin, S.M. (1991) Occupational therapy service: individual and collective understandings of the founders, part 1. *American Journal of Occupational Therapy*, **45**(4), 352–60.

Pioch, N. (1995) Romanticism. *WebMuseum, Paris*. http://www.ibiblio.org/wm/paint/glo/romanticism/ (17 March 2002).

Plewes, L.W. (1951) Modern treatment of fractures, with particular emphasis on the rehabilitation aspect. *Occupational Therapy*, **14**(2), 64–6.

Reilly, M. (1962) Eleanor Clarke Slagle Lecture: Occupational therapy can be one of the great ideas of 20th century medicine. *American Journal of Occupational Therapy*, **16**, 1–9.

Rivett, A. (1938/39) Fabric printing. *Journal of the Occupational Therapists' Association*, **1**(Winter), 19–22.

Rose, A. (1999) Spirituality and palliative care: the attitudes of occupational therapists. *British Journal of Occupational Therapy*, **62**, 307–12.

Ruskin, J. (1849) *The Seven Lamps of Architecture*, George Allen, London.

Ruskin, J. (1964) *The Stones of Venice*. Volume II. Series *Ruskin Today* (ed. K. Clark), John Murray, London (original work published 1853).

Russell, J.I. (1938) *The Occupational Treatment of Mental Illness*, Baillière, Tindall & Cox, London.

Saiedi, N. (1993) *The Birth of Social Theory: Social Thought in the Enlightenment and Romanticism*, Addison-Wesley Publishing Co., New York.

Schmid, T. (2005) *Promoting Health through Creativity: For Professionals in Health, Arts and Education*, John Wiley & Sons, New York.

Serrett, K.D. (1985) Another look at occupational therapy's history: paradigm or pair-of-hands? *Occupational Therapy in Mental Health*, **5**(3), 1–31.

Severn, E. (1951) Emotional education. *Occupational Therapy*, **14**(3), 112–16.

Sicely, M. (1950) Post-leucotomy rehabilitation. *Occupational Therapy*, **13**(1), 6–11.

Smith, M.D. (1945) Occupational therapy in a spinal injury centre. *Journal of the Association of Occupational Therapists*, **8**(Spring), 14–16.

Spencer, J., Davidson, H. and White, V. (1997) Helping clients develop hopes for the future. *American Journal of Occupational Therapy*, **51**(3), 191–8.

Spretnak, C. (1997) *The Resurgence of the Real: Body, Nature, and Place in a Hypermodern World*, Addison-Wesley Publishing Co., New York.

Stow, B.M. (1958) Occupational therapy in rehabilitation, in *Rehabilitation after Illness and Accident* (eds T.M. Ling and C.J.S. O'Malley), Baillière, Tindall & Cox, London, pp. 84–96.

Tarnas, R. (1996) *The Passion of the Western Mind: Understanding the Ideas that have Shaped our World View*, Pimlico, London.

Thornely, G. (1948) The rehabilitation of German wounded ex-servicemen: a British Red Cross scheme. *Journal of the Association of Occupational Therapists*, **11**(July), 21–5.

Toomey, M.A. (1999) The art of observation: reflecting on a spiritual moment. *Canadian Journal of Occupational Therapy*, **66**, 197–9.

Townsend, E. (2002) *Enabling Occupation: An Occupational Therapy Perspective*, revised edn, Canadian Association of Occupational Therapists, Ottawa.

Unruh, A.M., Versnel, J. and Kerr, N. (2002) Spirituality unplugged: a review of commonalities and contentions, and a resolution. *Canadian Journal of Occupational Therapy*, **69**(1), 5–19.

Wilcock, A.A. (2002) *Occupation for Health. Volume II: A Journey from Prescription to Self Health*, British Association and College of Occupational Therapists, London.

Yerxa, E.J. (1998) Health and the human spirit for occupation. *American Journal of Occupational Therapy*, **52**(6), 412–18.

Occupation for occupational therapists: how far will we go?

3

Clare Hocking and Ellen Nicholson

Introduction

In 2004, a text entitled *Occupation for Occupational Therapists* hit the professional bookshelves. Edited by Matthew Molineux, its basic premise was to bridge the gap between occupational science and occupational therapy practice. Described as a text for students and interested clinicians, the various chapters explore both conceptual issues around the nature of occupation and clinical issues around the implementation of occupation-based practice. Reflecting on the need for a book such as this, Molineux suggested that much of contemporary occupational therapy practice is 'a labour in vain' (p. 1). In supporting this claim he highlighted an outdated focus on impairment and performance components, which may be resolved by returning to a more traditional primary focus on occupation and health. While additional chapters explore topics such as occupational diagnosis, flow, pretend play, occupational reconstruction and population health and policy issues, the primary focus throughout is 'occupation for occupational therapists'.

In the brief discussion that follows, we explore two radical positions in relation to basing occupational therapy practice in occupation. In essence we ask, 'How far will we go?' What is the logical conclusion of recognising that occupation is not only the unique knowledge base, but also 'the means and the ends' of occupational therapy (Gray, 1998)? Two propositions are explored. The first is that occupation is *for occupational therapists*. Here, we take the standpoint that the knowledge generated by occupational science is the sole preserve of occupational therapists and question whether other professions can use that knowledge.

The second, with somewhat different emphasis, is that *occupation* is for occupational therapists. From this perspective, we ponder what we are implying when we call ourselves hand therapists, paediatric therapists or specialists in driving assessments. Are we not all occupation specialists? To begin the discussion, we turn to the first proposition.

A science of occupation

At the dawn of occupational science, it was held out to be a 'unique knowledge base' (Wilcock, 1991, p. 297), the foundation that would 'support the practice of occupational therapy' (Yerxa et al., 1990, p. 2). Under the auspices of this emerging science, people's 'need for and capacity to engage in and orchestrate daily occupations in the environment over the lifespan' (Yerxa et al., p. 6) would be revealed. 'Putting occupation under the microscope' (Wilcock, 1991, p. 298) would also expose its complex nature, show the effects of engaging in and being deprived of occupation, and explain the 'human striving for occupational competence and mastery' (Wilcock, 1991, p. 297). The 'rules, moral convictions, symbolic meanings . . . and sociocultural and historical contexts' (Clark et al., 1991, p. 302) that influence occupational choices would also be explored. Furthermore, what was learned would be organised into complex systems models. They would address such diverse perspectives as the biologically programmed aspects of occupation and the will to act. The experience of occupational engagement would be set alongside the cognitive processes involved, and the ways in which people's occupations are planned and organised would be considered within their social contexts (Clark et al., 1991; Yerxa et al., 1990).

Building this science, it was envisioned, would underline the profession's 'profound importance . . . to society' (Yerxa et al., 1990, p. 14). Indeed, the vision articulated by its founders was that occupational science would speak to important issues including the growing number of people who derive no enjoyment from their work, youth suicide, the drug epidemic and people unable to 'cope with the demands of daily living' (Yerxa et al., 1990, p. 3). It would also address the plight of people with a health condition, impairment, advancing age or some other circumstance that means their satisfaction with living is not assured. Armed with new understandings of these social ills, occupational therapists would justify the significance of their profession and differentiate it from others, to become 'more effective advocates for, and allies with people' with a disability (Yerxa et al., 1990, p. 3). Along the way, occupational therapy might become better understood by the public, the government, educational institutions and other health workers and, perhaps foremost in our minds, be freed from the requirement to follow medical prescriptions (Wilcock, 1991).

From the outset, it was expected that occupational science would draw from the 'array of disciplines' (Yerxa *et al.*, 1990, p. 6) that address aspects of occupation, including the biological and social sciences. That said, it alone would systematise and expand on this knowledge, to encompass 'the entire range of phenomena surrounding human occupation' (Clark *et al.*, 1991, p. 304). For while it would draw on interdisciplinary knowledge, the singular purpose of this new scientific discipline was to serve occupational therapy's future, to give it a scientific basis from which to work for the good of society (Clark *et al.*, 1991). This was a profession-centric view. None imagined that the knowledge of occupation that would be accumulated would inform other health professions. Occupational science was for occupational therapists.

Occupation for everyone?

Yet, alongside the renaissance of occupation that has welled up in occupational therapy (Whiteford *et al.*, 2000), there has been an observable upsurge of thinking about occupation in other quarters. Most notable is the World Health Organization's International Classification of Functioning, Disability and Health (ICF; WHO, 2001). The ICF proposes a dynamic relationship between health conditions, impairments to bodily structures and functions and participation in basic functions such as walking, as well as self-care, domestic, school, work and other facets of life. Personal factors, such as age, sex, life experience, fitness and ability to cope, and physical, material, social, attitudinal and institutional aspects of the environment are also identified as influential.

This linking of the personal, the environmental and participation within a model that addresses health and health outcomes mirrors the 'person-environment-occupation model' proposed within occupational therapy (Law *et al.*, 1996; Strong *et al.*, 1999). Not surprisingly, personal, environmental and occupational factors are also the key elements of Yerxa and colleagues' (1990) specifications for a science of occupation and Clark and colleagues' (1991) 'model of the human subsystems that influence occupation'. Thus, the elements that occupational therapists and occupational scientists brought together to establish a unique knowledge base have appeared, a decade later and with somewhat different emphasis, as key components of the ICF.

The World Health Organization's acknowledgement of the relationship between health conditions, activity and participation can be interpreted as a vindication of everything occupational therapists hold dear. At last, all health professions are charged with understanding the occupational impact of a health condition and gauging the value of their assessments, interventions and research agenda in terms of occupation or, in ICF terms, participation. The very thing we have battled to give legitimacy is now proclaimed to be the objective of health care services. Moreover, this demand comes from the highest quarter and at the insistence of people with disability, who require more than preservation of their lives: they want, as we all do, a life worth living.

With engagement in occupation reframed as participation and presented to health professions across the board, things have begun to move quickly. A quick scan of the professional literature readily shows that discussions about participation are under way in medicine, health promotion, nursing, physiotherapy and speech and language therapy, to name a few. Some authors have focused on how the ICF can inform their understanding of the ways that impairments impact on individuals' lives. One article, for example, brings together knowledge of the neurological disorders underlying cognitive disability, the impact that cognitive impairment has on major life areas, such as employment, and environmental solutions such as memory aids, spell checkers and safety alarms (Arthanat *et al.*, 2004). Others describe the disability that people experience in their everyday lives when they have disorders such as migraine (Leonardi *et al.*, 2005) or Alzheimer's disease (Muo *et al.*, 2005). Viewed from this perspective, new insights into the impact of health conditions have been generated, such as recognising that people with chronic back pain experience higher levels of disablement if their symptoms are less specific compared with those whose symptoms are more specific (Wormgoor *et al.*, 2006).

The ICF has also been used as a benchmark against which to critique established theories and to identify ways in which they might be extended to include factors promoting or impinging on participation in aspects of everyday life, such as employment and physical activity (Heerkens *et al.*, 2004; van der Ploeg *et al.*, 2004). Conversely, consistency between established assessment tools and the ICF has been claimed to validate their use in practice (Noreau *et al.*, 2004), while lack of consistency demonstrates the need to use existing assessments with caution and to develop assessments that more adequately address aspects of participation and environmental barriers (Sigl *et al.*, 2006).

Further applications of the ICF include attempts to ensure that health professionals address the participation outcomes espoused by the World Health Organization. Understanding the challenges that people experience is the first step towards determining outcomes, such as the South African physiotherapists who investigated using the ICF to document function and disability among people with HIV (Jelsma *et al.*, 2006). Speech and language therapists have also thought about how the ICF might be used to orchestrate a shift within their profession from focusing on the reduction of impairments to identifying participation goals. An example would be framing the goal as successfully communicating with peers rather than correctly pronouncing words (McLeod and Bleile, 2004). Others have examined the match between identified rehabilitation goals and ICF categories.

One such article cross-referenced rehabilitation goals, such as resuming dancing, managing the 'ironing, hanging the clothes up, cleaning, shopping and cooking' and working on the computer with the ICF participation categories of recreation and leisure, lifting and carrying objects, doing housework, fine hand use and remunerative employment (Cieza and Stucki, 2004, p. 150).

The ICF has also been employed as a yardstick of good practice which, by definition, is practice that achieves participation as well as medical outcomes. For example, one article identified the limitations of medical interventions that narrowly focus on biological processes (Shaw and Mackinnon, 2004). In the case study cited, the health team failed to recognise that occupations such as eating and walking can influence health outcomes. Because of this shortcoming, they overlooked the fact that the patient's diet lacked the vitamins associated with healing and his manner of walking put pressure on the open wounds on his toes. A more extreme example is the nurse educators who, inspired by the ICF's portrayal of the relationships between health, environment and participation, roundly criticised their profession for being too narrowly focused on medical diagnoses and thus failing to address activity limitations and participation restrictions (Kearney and Pryor, 2004).

Furthermore, perhaps stimulated by the ICF, physiotherapists in particular have turned their attention to the ways that participating in occupation affects people's physical status. Thus, researchers at the School of Physiotherapy in West Australia examined differences in strength and range of motion at the hip of female ballet dancers and non-dancers. Predictably, they measured anatomical differences, which they attributed to ballet training, as well as patterns of muscle development and lack of flexibility that they linked with risk of injury (Gupta et al., 2004). Similarly, physiotherapy researchers in New Zealand examined the magnitude of the spinal forces involved in shearing sheep and the extent to which commercially available back-support harnesses reduced those forces (Milosavljevic et al., 2004).

As this discussion shows, occupation or, for those informed by the ICF, participation, is being discussed in a multitude of contexts. This is not really surprising for, as Wilcock (2001) convincingly portrayed in the first volume of her history of occupational therapy, the relationship between health and the things people do has long been recognised. Acknowledging this, it would be naive in the extreme to claim that occupation is the sole preserve of occupational therapists. Clearly, others also legitimately claim to contribute to occupational outcomes.

But what of occupational science? Having recognised that this new field of knowledge development will be informed by interdisciplinary perspectives, are we comfortable with the thought that others might benefit from and apply the insights it generates? Can we, or perhaps should we, restrict our growing knowledge of occupation to occupational therapists?

This suggestion, clearly, is absurd. Just as occupational therapy has been informed by biology, medicine, psychology, sociology and so forth, occupational science will usefully inform others. Moreover, if the World Health Organization is to be successful in bringing participation to the fore of all health interventions, we might argue that all professions need to be informed by occupational science. But will they really understand it? Don't you need to be an occupational therapist to comprehend both the subtleties and the fundamental truths revealed by occupational science?

From our experiences of teaching the complexities of occupation to physiotherapists and podiatrists, we can attest that this is not the case. On the contrary, insights stimulated by occupational science, into the personal, social, cultural and historical meanings of occupation, intrigue and make sense to members of these professions as much as they intrigue occupational therapists new to this knowledge. What is more, we have observed not just the acquisition of new knowledge but also the translation of occupational knowledge into the context of physiotherapy and podiatry practice. For instance, one postgraduate physiotherapy student investigated the manual handling demands of mothering infants from psychosocial and environmental perspectives. The realities of slippery bath-time babies, tetchy babies who demand hours of comforting, treks to and from the car park carrying baby and the groceries, and the power of culturally entrenched values about being a loving mother, were acknowledged. The upshot was enriched understandings of why injuries occur, why mothers disregard advice about protecting their backs, shoulders and hands and the development of an occupationally focused line of questioning into the frequency, duration and biomechanical load of lifting, feeding, carrying, changing, transporting, comforting and playing with an infant.

Another physiotherapy student took her newfound knowledge of occupation back to the school where she works. She used it to rethink what was achieved in traditional physiotherapy practice, compared with what might be achieved if she used her skills to support children's participation in playground games and physical education classes. Significant here is the way that an occupational perspective led to new practice decisions about how to balance interventions to improve or preserve body structures and functions, against opportunities to engrain a pattern and expectation of participation in physical occupations that might sustain physical health over the child's lifetime.

But, does willingly sharing the profession's unique knowledge with members of other professions cast us as thieves, selling the family silver to earn our livelihood? We think not. At worst we are realists, acknowledging that occupational science findings are already in the public domain for all to see. More so, we are hopeful that occupational science will assist and inform all health professionals in their journey towards realising the World Health Organization's vision. We are also confident, based on experience thus far, that studying occupational science does not turn physiotherapists or podiatrists into occupational therapists, or people who try to do our job. Developing a depth of understanding of occupation, and what motivates, shapes, enables and constrains it, makes a better physiotherapist, nurse, doctor, gerontologist, speech and language therapist, counsellor or community developer. In introducing other professions to occupational science, we understand that it will indeed serve society, albeit in ways not envisioned at the outset. So, occupation for occupational therapists? On balance: no, occupation for everyone.

Occupational therapy specialists

If occupation is for all, where does that leave us as occupational therapists? More particularly, how does it position us in the face of the realities of clinical governance and tighter legislation around competence for practice? In New Zealand, for example, the Health Practitioners Competence Assurance Act (2003) requires all registered health practitioners, every year, to provide evidence of their competence. This is just one instance in an international trend that means that evidence-based practice will be the way of the future. Acknowledging this, we can identify that the unique body of evidence that informs occupational therapy practice is our specialist knowledge and therapeutic use of occupation.

Yet, as a profession we continue to struggle with recognising and proclaiming this specialty. This is never more evident than when we slip away from calling ourselves 'occupational therapists'. Think of paediatric therapists, visiting neurodevelopmental therapists, driving assessors and hand therapists, to name but a few. These titles name occupational therapists (and other related professionals) according to their specialist context of practice. Moreover, in privileging therapists with these titles, we reward them for having specialist knowledge in a particular clinical area. But is this not confusing the issue . . . specialist knowledge of what? And specialist according to whom?

The case against specialisms: When is an occupational therapist not an occupational therapist?

As noted above, there is a tendency within occupational therapy to reward therapists who have demonstrated expertise in a particular skill, such as driving assessment, or who have advanced knowledge in an identified clinical area, such as paediatrics, with a specialist title. This title is added to their qualifications, or replaces their professional title. One example of this is the American Occupational Therapy Association certification initiatives, in the course of which practising therapists and association members were surveyed. The outcome was that 'external factors' (namely, need in society, increased value of certification, legislative-regulatory issues and availability of literature and resources) were identified as determining two levels of specialist certification (Glantz, 2003, p. 11).

The first level, specialty certification, is awarded based on competency and recognises practice specialties relevant to the scope of occupational therapy that possess a defined set of skills, techniques and interventions (Glantz, 2003). These have been confirmed to be: driver rehabilitation and community mobility; cognition; environmental modification; feeding and swallowing; and low vision (Glantz, 2004). The second, board certification, is awarded following a 'rigorous self study process' (p. 11). It is an advanced practice designation for occupational therapists experienced in a major area of occupational therapy practice (Glantz, 2003): paediatrics; gerontology; mental health; and physical rehabilitation (Glantz, 2004). Sceptics among us might even argue that our American colleagues are the true holders of specialist knowledge, particularly as more and more specialisms are added to the certification process over time.

But where does it end? This trend towards increasing numbers of specialisms within the profession is alarming for a number of reasons, primarily the apparent lack of philosophical discussion and debate around what it means to be the holder of specialist knowledge. More specifically, there is a lack of agreement around what the specialist knowledge might actually be, and an apparent lack of international standardisation of recognised specialisms. Reviewing the issues raises so many more questions than answers: Who governs the process of developing specialisms? Who is responsible for determining the level at which a specialist must demonstrate specialist skills? Is 'rigorous self study' truly indicative of specialist knowledge and skills? What skills and knowledge are expected of a specialist? Is there a clear relationship between practising within a recognised specialism and competence for practice? What does working with an occupational therapist who is a specialist mean to our clients, and does this status influence their expectations of therapists? An important corollary is: how do we, and our clients, regard occupational therapists who are not specialists?

Despite giving rise to such awkward questions, the trend towards increasing specialisms is surprisingly popular. Yet it flies in the face of everything we know about evidence-based practice. That is, claims of specialist practice dismiss the fact that there is a significant lack of reputable and conclusive evidence for a number of interventions and approaches utilised in everyday occupational therapy practice, let alone in specialist practice areas. What we do know about the application of evidence in practice is that the evidence that addresses the core of occupational therapy practice is about occupation. In addition, describing specialist knowledge in terms of a practice context such as paediatrics, hand therapy or mental health is a reductionist, and often medically focused, way of approaching the issue of defining specialisms. Falling into the trap of having medically labelled specialisms denies the fact that occupational therapy has worked hard to distance itself from these paradigms.

Compared with the United States experience, the British Association and College of Occupational Therapists was more measured in its development of specialist sections. These are groups of occupational therapists with a common interest or similar area of employment, who are working in partnership with the College of Occupational Therapists (COT) to promote their area of clinical interest (COT, 2004). These sections include groups such as the College of Occupational Therapists Specialist Section – Mental Health, the College of Occupational Therapists Specialist Section – Independent Practice and the College of Occupational Therapists Specialist Section – HIV/AIDS, Oncology and Palliative Care. These sections are distinguished from special interest groups, which do not have formal recognition from the College. The difference? These therapists are occupational therapists first – then specialists in a particular area, knowledge or skill base.

Countering this debate, Fitzpatrick and Presnell (2004) would probably consider this argument against specialisms deeply flawed. In their article, entitled 'Can occupational therapists be hand therapists?' the adoption of the ICF as a framework to examine the consequences of hand injuries is proposed. In the context of their discussion, Fitzpatrick and Presnell appear to argue that professional titles are irrelevant. Instead, the interpretation of the title by the specialist (in this case, an occupational therapist with specialist knowledge in occupation and hand function) determines whether and how that title is relevant in a particular context. This argument for semantics offers an alternative perspective but fails to address the elitist message sent by recognising specialisms, and how the recipients of occupational therapy services, and other team members, might interpret that message. Furthermore, in the context of this discussion, it is deeply perplexing to be presented with the suggestion that occupation might at times be irrelevant to an occupational therapist's practice.

Identifying the specialist knowledge of occupational therapists: the link between theory and practice

While a number of theorists and clinicians have steadfastly maintained the centrality of occupation in occupational therapy practice, a recent development in the literature hails a return to this very premise. Drawing on the ICF, Coster (1998) described the importance of a top-down approach to assessing children. In this, she encouraged therapists to identify occupational performance issues rather than impairments as a point of entry with clients.

Coster is not alone. Respected authors such as Law *et al.* (2001) support the notion that an occupation-based perspective is currently lacking from conceptual models of occupation, which do not address developmental influences, and from developmental approaches to paediatric practice, which tend to focus on assessment and remediation of sensory and motor impairments. Responding to similar concerns, Polatajko *et al.* (2000) developed their 'dynamic performance analysis', a process that combines assessment and intervention to directly address occupational performance issues.

Supporting these initiatives towards occupationally focused assessments, interventions and ways of viewing clients are the recently developed models of practice that focus on occupational performance. One such, the 'cognitive orientation to occupational performance model' (CO-OP; Missiuna *et al.*, 2001), draws on a wealth of knowledge of occupation. In explicitly drawing from this knowledge, however, it directly challenges therapists to review traditional, and often poorly evidenced, approaches to paediatric practice.

Developments such as this are not, of course, always welcomed. A bemused year 3 occupational therapy student recently witnessed senior therapists leaving the room during her presentation of the phenomenal outcomes for children she had worked with using the CO-OP approach. They were apparently disinterested in this 'non-traditional' and, in their eyes inappropriate, approach to therapy (J. Hornell, personal communication, 14 November 2004).

Where to from here?

In this chapter, we have pondered what occupation for occupational therapists really means. While we acknowledge that others will have different points of view, our foundational belief is that occupation is both the means and the ends of occupational therapy. It is our principal focus, what we do and what we aspire to achieve. While we have argued on pragmatic and client-centred grounds that knowledge of occupation must be shared with other professions, we are secure in asserting that this will in no way undermine occupational therapy as a profession. Our confidence in making this claim is founded on an understanding that where occupation is this profession's primary therapeutic tool, other professions have their own, equally valued tools. For them occupation, or participation, is just part of the information they seek about the genesis, progression and impact of illness, injury or injustice. Occupation is merely the goal or end point of their intervention.

However, while we profess a high level of comfort with sharing the growing knowledge of occupation with others, we suggest that uncomfortable questions will arise as the profession's reawakening to occupation proceeds. Our focus in this regard has been on the consequences of fully owning occupation as the core of our knowledge for specialist areas of practice. Driving assessment apart, the specialisms we commonly identify align with medical rather than occupational conceptions of the world. Identifying such specialisms within occupational therapy, we maintain, is of central concern. Accordingly, we have argued for an end to recognising specialisms derived from biomedical populations, health conditions or areas of dysfunction. Yet our position in relation to specialisms is not clear-cut, in that we have asserted that occupational therapists cannot and should not continue to privilege existing specialty areas of practice, while suggesting that the profession can and should recognise specialist knowledge of occupation.

Our position, therefore, is that occupational therapy needs to begin again with an international forum to discuss and debate further the questions and concerns raised by specialist practice areas. We believe that there needs to be a clearly articulated philosophy around the purpose and value of specialisms in the context of contemporary practice. Such a discussion would need to include standardising the specialist knowledge required to work in identified specialist areas. It may be that something as simple as changing the way that occupational therapists describe their specialties would address some of these issues.

That said, we believe that occupational therapists are first and foremost *occupation* therapists. The profession's specialist knowledge lies in recognising the value of occupation in the lives of its clients and in the use of occupation as a therapeutic tool. Following this line of reasoning, a paediatric occupational therapist becomes an occupational therapist with specialist knowledge in childhood occupations. A little wordier, granted, but a more accurate representation of the therapist's specialist knowledge base. Perhaps most important, specialisms thus named recognise the direction of the profession, the value of evidence in practice and the unique nature of our very special knowledge; occupation.

Acknowledgements

Sections of this discussion started their life as an assignment completed in partial fulfilment of the requirements for the Doctor of Health Science from Auckland University of Technology, New Zealand.

References

Arthanat, S., Nochajski, S.M. and Stone, J. (2004) The international classification of functioning, disability and health and its application to cognitive disorder. *Disability and Rehabilitation*, **26**(4), 235–45.

Cieza, A. and Stucki, G. (2004) New approaches to understanding the impact of musculoskeletal conditions. *Best Practice and Research: Clinical Rheumatology*, **18**(2), 141–54.

Clark, F.A., Parham, D., Carlson, M.E., Frank, G., Jackson, J., Pierce, D., Wolfe, R.J. and Zemke, R. (1991) Occupational science: academic innovation in the service of occupational therapy's future. *American Journal of Occupational Therapy*, **45**(4), 300–10.

College of Occupational Therapists (2004) Specialist sections. www.cot.org.uk/specialist/intro.php (20 December 2004).

Coster, W. (1998) Occupation-centred assessment of children. *American Journal of Occupational Therapy*, **52**(5), 337–44.

Fitzpatrick, N. and Presnell, S. (2004) Can occupational therapists be hand therapists? *British Journal of Occupational Therapy*, **67**(11), 508–10.

Glantz, C. (2003) Update on AOTA certification initiatives. *OT Practice*, 15 December 2003, 11.

Glantz, C. (2004) Recommendations for AOTA certification programs. *OT Practice*, 10 May 2004, 9–10.

Gray, J. (1998) Putting occupation into practice: occupation as ends, occupation as means. *American Journal of Occupational Therapy*, **52**(5), 354–64.

Gupta, A., Fernihough, B., Bailey, G., Bombeck, P., Clarke, A. and Hopper, D. (2004) An evaluation of differences in hip external rotation strength and range of motion between female dancers and non-dancers. *British Journal of Sports Medicine*, **38**(6), 778–83.

Health Practitioners Competency Assurance Act (2003) Wellington: New Zealand Government.

Heerkens, Y., Engels, J., Kuiper, C., van der Gulden, J. and Oostendorp, R. (2004) The use of the ICF to describe work related factors influencing the health of employees. *Disability and Rehabilitation*, **26**(17), 1060–6.

Jelsma, J., Brauer, N., Hahn, C., Snoek, A. and Sykes, I. (2006) A pilot study to investigate the use of the ICF in documenting levels of function and disability in people living with HIV. *South African Journal of Physiotherapy*, **62**(1), 7–13.

Kearney, P.M. and Pryor, J. (2004) The International Classification of Functioning, Disability and Health (ICF) and nursing. *Journal of Advanced Nursing*, **46**(2), 162–70.

Law, M., Cooper, B., Strong, S., Stewart, D., Rigby, P. and Letts, L. (1996) The person-environment-occupation model: a transactive approach to occupational performance. *Canadian Journal of Occupational Therapy*, **63**, 9–23.

Law, M., Missiuna, C., Pollock, N. and Stewart, D. (2001) Foundations for occupational therapy practice for children, in *Occupational Therapy for Children*, 4th edn (ed. J. Case-Smith), Mosby, St Louis, MO, pp. 39–70.

Leonardi, M., Steiner, T.J., Scher, A.T. and Lipton, R.B. (2005) The global burden of migraine: measuring disability in headache disorders with WHO's Classification of Functioning, Disability and Health (ICF). *Journal of Headache and Pain*, **6**(6), 429–40.

McLeod, S. and Bleile, K. (2004) The ICF: a framework for setting goals for children with speech impairment. *Child Language Teaching and Therapy*, **20**(3), 199–219.

Milosavljevic, S., Carman, A.B., Milburn, P.D., Wilson, B.D. and Davidson, P.L. (2004) The influence of a back support harness on spinal forces during sheep shearing. *Ergonomics*, **47**(11), 1208–25.

Missiuna, C., Mandich, A., Polatajko, H. and Malloy-Miller, T. (2001) Cognitive orientation to daily occupational performance (CO-OP): Part 1: Theoretical foundations. *Physical and Occupational Therapy in Pediatrics*, **29**, 69–81.

Molineux, M. (ed.) (2004) *Occupation for Occupational Therapists*. Blackwell Publishing Ltd, Oxford, UK.

Muo, R., Schindler, A., Vernero, I., Schindler, O., Ferrario, E. and Frisoni, G.B. (2005) Alzheimer's disease-associated disability: an ICF approach. *Disability and Rehabilitation*, **27**(23), 1405–13.

Noreau, L., Desrosiers, J., Robichaud, L., Fougeyrollas, P., Rochette, A. and Viscogliosi, C. (2004) Measuring social participation: reliability of the LIFE-H in older adults with disabilities. *Disability and Rehabilitation*, **26**(6), 346–52.

Polatajko, H.J., Mandich, A. and Martini, R. (2000) Dynamic performance analysis: a framework for understanding occupational performance. *American Journal of Occupational Therapy*, **54**(1), 65–72.

Shaw, L. and Mackinnon, J. (2004) A multidimensional view of health. *Education for Health: Change in Learning and Practice*, **17**(2), 213–22.

Sigl, T., Cieza, A., Brockow, T., Chatterji, S., Kostanjsek, N. and Stucki, G. (2006) Content comparison of low back pain-specific measures based on the International Classification of Functioning, Disability and Health (ICF). *Clinical Journal of Pain*, **22**(2), 147–53.

Strong, S., Rigby, P., Stewart, D., Law, M., Letts, L. and Cooper, B. (1999) Application of the Person-Environment-Occupation Model: a practical tool. *Canadian Journal of Occupational Therapy*, **66**, 122–33.

Van der Ploeg, H.P., van der Beek, A.J., van der Woude, L.H.V. and van Mechelen, W. (2004) Physical activity for people with a disability. *Sports Medicine*, **34**(10), 639–49.

Whiteford, G., Townsend, E. and Hocking, C. (2000) Reflections on a renaissance of occupation. *Canadian Journal of Occupational Therapy*, **67**(1), 61–9.

Wilcock, A. (1991) Occupational science. *British Journal of Occupational Therapy*, **54**(8), 297–300.

Wilcock, A.A. (2001) *Occupation for Health. Volume 1: A Journey from Self Health to Prescription*. British Association and College of Occupational Therapists, London.

World Health Organization (2001) *International Classification of Functioning, Disability and Health*. World Health Organization, Geneva.

Wormgoor, M.E.A., Indahl, A., van Tulder, M.W. and Kemper, H.C.G. (2006) Functioning description according to the ICF model in chronic back pain: disablement appears even more complex with decreasing symptom-specificity. *Journal of Rehabilitation Medicine*, **38**(2), 93–9.

Yerxa, E.J., Clark, F., Frank, G., Jackson, J., Parham, D., Pierce, D., Stein, C. and Zemke, R. (1990) An introduction to occupational science: a foundation for occupational therapy in the 21st century. *Occupational Therapy in Health Care*, **6**(4), 1–17.

A psychoanalytic discourse in occupational therapy

4

Lindsey Nicholls

Introduction

'It is only with the heart that one can see rightly;
what is essential is invisible to the eye.'

(*The Little Prince*, De Saint-Exupery, 1974, p. 70)

Psychoanalysis, rather than an archaic language that refers to mankind's predetermined sexual drives and/or perversions, speaks to the heart of what it means to be human. Any serious study of the analytic theories and theorists will reassure occupational therapists that they are probably already somewhat aware (if not fully cognisant) of the emotional significance within the concepts, either inside the experience of their own lives or as they have come to understand the life world of their clients. Psychoanalysis is a language of understanding one's feelings through the process of thinking, a process that I have termed 'being concerned with matters of the heart'.

Craib, a sociologist and psychoanalyst, has written a very accessible text on psychoanalysis (2001), from which I have drawn heavily in this chapter, but it is his earlier book, *The Importance of Disappointment* (1994), that so eloquently speaks to the heart of the matter. He writes the book after he has been diagnosed with cancer, and so the book's introduction, as quoted below, is particularly poignant as the reader can feel he is talking about himself but within his words we recognise ourselves.

I had never before allowed myself to recognise the fear of death that must be common to us all, and neither had I properly understood its implications:

that life is immensely precious and the links we have with people, in all their dreadful complexity, are all that we have, and if there is such a thing as evil it lies in the deliberate breaking of those links . . . there is much about our modern world that increases disappointment and at the same time encourages us to hide from it: to act as if what is good in life does not entail the bad – for example, that we can love and be loved by another person without having to give up other aspects of our lives; that we can have children without sacrifice; that we can love without ambivalence and hatred; that we can take decisions about our lives without being bounded on all sides by the needs and actions of others; that we can grow without the pain and loss, and in the end we can grow without dying.

(Craib, 1994,p. vii)

It has seemed that, in recent years, occupational therapists have pursued professional credibility through their allegiance to models of practice espoused by modern (current) proponents of an occupational therapy and/or science theory (Christiansen and Baum, 1997; Fearing and Clark, 2000; Kielhofner, 1995; Townsend, 1997; Zemke and Clark, 1996) – and that what has been neglected is the early contribution of psychoanalysis to the profession. A psychoanalytic view of activity and the therapeutic relationship, which was promoted in the early work of Fidler and Fidler (1963), has been subsumed by authors who maintain a view of the world that is wholly conscious, socially and/or culturally motivated and responsive to clear explanations and good intentions.

Perhaps the most profound loss in our current discourse has been an appreciation of the unconscious and the effect that it can have on the actions and choices of individuals and within society. In the current climate of evidence-based practice and measurable outcomes that are reliant on positivist views of science and therapy, there has been a loss of wonder and delight in (appreciation of) the imaginative potential of the unconscious with its capacity to repair, reconcile and recover. The unconscious carries within it not only instinctual drives, and their concomitant anxiety, but also a capacity for connection, knowledge, wisdom and creativity (Banks and Blair, 1997; Fidler and Fidler, 1963, 1978; Milner, 1999; Segal, 1986).

I think that what is valuable in Freud, and the psychoanalytic theorists who followed him, is the always implicit, sometimes explicit, message that we can never quite be what we want to be.

(Craib, 1994, p. 35)

Freud has been considered the 'father' of all known forms of psychotherapy (Brown and Peddar, 1991); he did not invent psychotherapy (Bateman and Holmes, 1995) but was able to articulate a formal theory of the human psyche alongside a description of a therapy that could alleviate the suffering of people who had mental (emotional) difficulties. This form of help, psychotherapy, is in its essence a 'talking cure' (Brown and Peddar, 1991, p. 11) and its basic tenets are shared among all the psychotherapies – those in which the therapist establishes a relationship with a patient (known as the client, in humanistic schools of thought) in order for the patient to explore their inner lives and circumstances that contributed to their unhappiness (or 'dis-ease' with themselves). In understanding themselves, clients are able to engage more fully in relationships with others and contribute to their world through meaningful work (or occupations).

Occupational therapists have been cognisant of the work of psychotherapy and have incorporated into their practice many of the techniques used by the emergent psychotherapies, such as the use of anxiety management training techniques, which are derived from the cognitive behavioural therapists.

Psychoanalysis is one branch (albeit the central theory or root from which other psychotherapies and theories emerged) of psychotherapy, and its distinguishing features (in an area where there is much overlap, debate and discussion) are its belief in the unconscious, the role of early childhood experiences as providing fundamental structures for the personality and the importance of transference and countertransference in the client's relationship with the therapist (Bateman and Holmes, 1995). Occupational therapists have seemingly kept away from these areas of interest in recent years – in my opinion, to the detriment of the profession – in occupational therapy any idea or acknowledgement of the role of the unconscious in our work has itself become unconscious. This may have been due to the rise in interest in the more pragmatic and action-orientated methods used by (for example) cognitive behavioural therapists. These approaches may have appeared to be more in keeping with the focus on activity by occupational therapists – but it has meant the loss of curiosity (wonder) in the process of creativity and a loss of focus in, and thereby a devaluing of, the relationship with the client.

Psychoanalytic theory gives us an understanding of people and their relationships with themselves and others, as well as the occupations in which they invest time and interest. This can offer occupational therapists an awareness of, and way of working with, clients that is rewarding and enriching. At the same time, psychoanalytic theory can make us (client and therapist) more aware of our vulnerabilities and of our ongoing struggle to be honest with ourselves and concerned for the well-being of others.

The purpose of this chapter

I have had an interest in and involvement with a psychoanalytic view of occupational therapy for so much of my professional life that I can no longer see clearly without these conceptual lenses. (The idea of theory (structure) being used as a lens through which to view the world – 'a pair of spectacles with a specially tinted filter' – comes from Hagedorn, 1992, p. 14.) This frame of reference has influenced how I have engaged with clients and understood their choice of occupations, and it has helped me to reflect on my relationships with colleagues and multidisciplinary team members within the context of care. It is a concern to me that over the past 40 years a psychoanalytic discourse in occupational therapy has almost completely disappeared from our professional literature, except for a few lone and brave voices (Banks and Blair, 1997; Cole, 1998; Collins, 2004; Daniel and Blair, 2002a, b; Creek, 1997b; Hagedorn, 1992). It is my wish to persuade occupational therapists to consider (or reconsider) what psychoanalysis can offer us in our endeavour to alleviate the suffering of our clients and support their sense of purpose in day-to-day life.

I am not proposing to (re)write a definition of what occupational therapists do, or even what occupation or activity mean, and I have no high-minded aim of creating a new theoretical model in occupational therapy. I do, however, hope to encourage occupational therapists to re-engage with psychoanalytic theory and practice as a way of understanding their clients and their experiences in doing the work of an occupational therapist. This chapter covers a brief description of the purpose of psychoanalysis within two main areas: occupations as (symbolic) representations of human needs, and the unconscious use of defences in organisations or professional cultures that can be unhelpful (anti-task).

The curious concept of occupation

In 1999, I was working as an occupational therapist on an inpatient drug rehabilitation facility. The therapeutic programme incorporated a daily early morning community meeting that aimed to establish a culture of co-operation and responsibility within the patient group, many of whom were feeling vulnerable from the physical effects of detoxification and, often, a personal sense of hopelessness, guilt and anger at themselves. I was a fairly new staff member when a client, who was known to many of the other staff from previous admissions, asked who I was. I said my name and added that I was an occupational therapist. The client, a 34-year-old pregnant woman, asked: 'What *is* an occupational therapist?'

Her tone was somewhat unfriendly, and I suspected that she already had an idea about my role, and so I somewhat playfully replied that it depended on what she thought an occupation was. She answered: 'I didn't ask you for a **** lecture, I asked you what you *did*.'

In a way, she expressed the exasperation that many of us feel in trying to explain what it is that we do, and the ever recurring and increasingly elaborate definitions of occupational therapy attest to that frustration. I have always found a quote by Reilly (1985) about the ordinariness of our interventions (that is, what we *do*) deeply reassuring:

> The wide and gaping chasm which exists between the complexity of illness and the commonplaceness of our treatment tools is, and always will be, both the pride and the anguish of our profession.
>
> (Reilly, 1985, p. 88)

The attempt to define occupation has occupied the profession for the past 20 years, prompted by a call to return to our philosophical and theoretical roots (e.g. Hasselkus, 2002; Wilcock, 1998a, 2001, 2002; Whiteford *et al.* 2000; Yerxa, 1998). The essence of occupation is difficult to capture because it is an empty category until the ideas of meaning, purpose and motivation are added to our understanding. On the surface, occupations can be descriptions that portray the external reality of doing, for example, fly-fishing, meditation or cooking maize meal. However, without examining the inner processes that drive a person to do a particular occupation, it remains only a possibility of doing – what I have called an empty category but one that we (as a profession) are very curious about.

Many recent authors have included the dimensions of meaning and motivation in books (Hasselkus, 2002) and research papers (Christiansen, 1999) and a new branch of study, that of occupational science, has developed to examine the notion of occupation (Zemke and Clark, 1996). Very few of these studies or papers carry the idea of the unconscious as contributing to an understanding of why people do what they do. In the next section I consider occupations as representing an unconscious need of the individual; this may be as a form of defence against vulnerability and a way of coping with existential anxiety or as a way of demonstrating a desire for reparative action through a creative endeavour.

A disavowal of dependency

> How much of the appeal of mountaineering lies in its simplification of inter-personal relationships, its reduction of friendship to smooth interaction (like war), its substitution of an other (the mountain, the challenge) for the relationship itself? Behind a mystique of adventure, toughness, footloose vagabondage – all much needed antidotes to our culture's built-in comfort and convenience – may lie a kind of adolescent refusal to take seriously aging, the frailty of others, interpersonal responsibility, weakness of all kinds, the slow unspectacular course of life itself.
>
> (Roberts, in Krakauer, 1997, p. 45)

Since my own modest but personally harsh experience of walking in the Himalayas (in 1995), I have been fascinated by written accounts of mountain climbing by the mountaineers themselves (Bonington, 2001; Krakauer, 1997; Simpson, 1997a, b), and by biographies of climbers who have died in their endeavours to conquer the world's highest mountains (for example, Douglas & Rose (2000). While reading such books, I came across the above quote and began to think about these physical endeavours as being a defense against the internal experience of human vulnerability.

It occurred to me that the occupation of mountain climbing has a compulsive quality. Climbers speak about having to go back to climbing mountains again and again, as Joe Simpson has done many times since his near fatal accident described in the book (1997a) and recent film (2004), *Touching the Void*. The compulsion to keep going onwards and upwards is sometimes despite other people who are in difficulty. Simpson (1997b) wrote a passionate diatribe against climbers who walk past those, less fortunate, who have collapsed in the extreme conditions and who cannot continue in their quest for the summit and may even die. This at-all-costs ambition seems to be evidence of the disavowal of a human need for connection with another, in other words, climbing is a substitute for real relationships. Indeed, it may be an unconscious defence against the experience of vulnerability or emotional dependence.

Object relations theory, which places the relationships we have with each other as the 'primary motivational drive' (Banks and Blair, 1997, p. 89), proposes that it is the very nature of this fundamental dependence and connection that we have with each other which causes us such inner conflict and turmoil. Segal (1997) said that a person's capacity to acknowledge and manage their connection to (reliance on) others is divided into two mechanisms, the manic defence and the desire for reparation. The manic defence is organised against any experience of need (vulnerability) or guilt, and the desire for reparation, which can 'lead to further growth of the ego' (p. 82) is often seen in a person's devotion to an action which results in a creative act (such as writing a book) or a work ambition (for example, joining Voluntary Service Overseas).

The difference in the two defence mechanisms (manic and reparative) is that the manic defence can be seen as a need to act that in its essence denies any experience of personal vulnerability or culpability. As such, it does not allow the individual to mature through an engagement with the other, as Joe Simpson (1997a) so poignantly describes a group of climbers huddling in a tent, denying the reality of a person lying outside in the bitter cold waving one arm. The climbers reassured themselves that they could not have saved him and that any effort to do so would deplete their resources, in other words, render them incapable of achieving their goal of reaching the summit.

If we are to explore the reasons why people do what they do, there is much to be gained by understanding the object relations school of thought in psychoanalysis. The founder member of this school was Melanie Klein (1882–1960), who based her theories on her analysis of children using a form of free association – play. Klein, in describing the two states of mind from which the infant develops and which continue to influence all adult experiences and relationships, the paranoid schizoid and depressive positions, examined the capacity an individual had for experiencing guilt (described in Segal, 1988).

Klein described how the infant initially experiences his or her world as being filled with good (feeding and comforting) objects (persons) and separate bad (withholding and punishing) objects, known as the paranoid schizoid position. This perception changes as the infant realises that the objects (good and bad) are one person (that is, the mother) and at that point the hateful and destructive feelings the infant has had towards the bad object are felt as threatening to overwhelm and destroy the very object who is able to nurture and protect the infant. It is at this point that the infant reaches the 'depressive position' – in other words, is able to perceive the 'whole' object and experience guilt at their destructive impulses. These unconscious feelings of fearing that the loved object is potentially destroyed by the infant's hatred (or envy) is defended against through the two mechanisms mentioned earlier – the manic defence and the reparative drive. In reading the accounts of mountaineers, I was struck by their similarity to the description of a manic defence:

> The infant discovers his dependence on his mother, his sense of valuing her and, together with this dependence, he discovers his ambivalence and experiences his intense feelings of rage and fear of loss, mourning, pining and guilt in relation to his object, external and internal. It is against this whole experience that the manic defense organization is directed. Since the depressive position is linked with the experience of dependence on the object, manic defenses will be directed against any feelings of dependence which will be obviated, denied or reversed.
>
> (Segal 1988, p. 83)

As occupational therapists, we may need to consider whether our focus on activities (or a desire for an activity) is a form of manic defensive when working with clients; the activity representing a substitute for an experience of an internal distress or unconscious fear of a destructive intent towards the client.

Object relations theorists, such as Klein, Winnicott and Bion (Craib, 2001), place relationships with others as central to all that we are and do in life. Their understanding of our dependence on others as a necessary and problematical part of us has much merit in occupational therapy theory. Craib (1994), in writing about the value of psychoanalysis, stated that 'dependence is inevitable, and of course it is inevitable not simply when we are very young or very old: it is necessary, and is a fact throughout our lives, economically, politically, physically and psychologically' (p. 187). There is much in our modern culture which denies this dependency (Hoggett, 2000) but on a deeper (psychic) level each person must struggle with feelings of dependency on others. This struggle can be expressed through choice of occupations, for example, using mountain climbing as an unconscious defence against an experience of dependency, or quilting a bed cover in a co-operative group activity as an expression of commitment to others (that is, a reparative engagement in an activity).

The idea of an occupation as a representation of unconscious needs and defences was evident in the work of Fidler and Fidler (1963), who drew our attention to the occupations chosen by the patient as potentially reinforcing 'their psychotic or neurotic defenses' (p. 74). They suggested that we need to analyse the patient's actions and choices in order to encourage different activities that can promote growth and maturity.

> An hypothesis exists that since action is the natural antidote for anxiety, any action or activity will relieve anxiety. It has been further hypothesized that the nature of the activity is far less important than the fact the patient is doing something. . . . Involvement in an activity can be either therapeutic or damaging to the patient, and therefore it is essential that we become more aware of and more carefully evaluate the psychodynamics of activities.
>
> (Fidler and Fidler, 1963, p. 72)

Many of the ideas in this original work show an understanding of psychoanalytic concepts and draw our attention to the symbolic content of occupations. Unfortunately, the authors move from interpreting the need some patients may have for what are termed 'regressive' activities to becoming highly prescriptive in recommending certain activities. In this prescriptive approach to pathology lies the problem with their theory. They suggest that by engaging in a different activity the person's inner turmoil will be alleviated and/or changed for the better. What the authors have ignored is that the choice of occupation is a symbolic representation of inner and outward processes and that changing the overt manifestation of this struggle will not change the impulse (drive) for the activity.

How can occupational therapists distinguish between occupations that enable the self to express its innermost needs and those that defend or deflect the self from the expression and fulfilment of those needs? Wilcock (in Hasselkus, 2002), a prolific and thoughtful writer about occupation and well-being, draws our attention to the fact that doing occupations 'may be injurious to health and well-being'

(p. 95). Her ideas, echoed by Hasselkus, help us as a profession to be more critical in understanding occupations. However, these authors do not consider the role of unconscious anxiety that may be driving the person to engage in activities that are 'injurious to health' and that may explain the compulsion to return to the same comforting state of risk.

> As a means of relaxing, climbing is unique. Whatever preoccupations a leader may have before starting the climb, within a short distance of leaving the ground they would have been pushed to the very back of the mind. It is the ultimate displacement activity . . . Being committed, whether it is on a fifty foot crag or a mountain wall two miles high, means going beyond the point where retreat is feasible, where it is almost certainly easier to go on up and reach the top than to climb back down.
>
> (Rose and Douglas, 1999, p. 30)

I am not suggesting that people who climb mountains are unbalanced individuals who should be offered a period of intensive psychotherapy to cure them of their need to place themselves in positions of high risk. I, alongside many others, celebrate their achievements and enjoy my own modest adventures. Rather, I am using their craving to climb a mountain as an opportunity to explore possible conscious and unconscious meanings as a way of understanding what is done and why it may be done.

To return to the story of the patent in the drug rehabilitation ward, who wanted to know what I *did*, I became aware of her inner distress and need to use drugs in a discussion we had shortly after the birth of her third child. She said that she found it unbearable to be with her baby because its cries made her feel empty. As she told me this, she began to cry and said that she had never been without drugs when she was with her other children. She said she needed to 'numb herself up' in order to be with them. She said the feeling inside her that they provoked with their cries was of 'the void'.

Other patients on the drug rehabilitation ward had described this experience (and fear) of an inner hollow that they expressed as 'the nothingness'. They said that they were terrified of this space, sometimes expressed as time, sometimes as the lack of meaningful occupation. The clients often said that they would use drugs to occupy their time; drug taking was their occupation, with its elaborate rituals, social connection and ultimate physical satisfaction.

These discussions about drugs and how they provide fulfilment helped me to make the link to the climbing literature. Joe Simpson's (1997b) moving account of his experience of extreme vulnerability following a fall, with his fear of dying alone in an ice chasm, can be read as an account of survival against the odds or as a description of existential anguish.

The tyranny of time

In his book, *The Curious Incident of Dog in the Night-Time*, Mark Haddon wrote as if he were a 15-year-old boy (Christopher) with Asperger's syndrome. He wrote a wonderful description of time.

> When I used to play with my train set I made a train timetable because I liked timetables. And I like timetables because I like to know when everything is going to happen. (p. 192)
>
> Because time is not like space. And when you put something down somewhere, like a protractor or a biscuit, you can have a map in your head to tell you where you have left it, but even if you don't have a map it will still be there because a map is a representation of things that actually exist so you can find the protractor or the biscuit again. And a timetable is a map of time, except that if you don't have a timetable time is not there like the landing and the garden *and* the route to school. Because time is only the relationship between the way different things change, like the earth going round the sun and atoms vibrating and clocks ticking and day and night and waking up and going to sleep. (p. 193)
>
> And this means that time is a mystery, and not even a thing, and no one has ever solved the puzzle of what time is, exactly. And so, if you get lost in time it is like being lost in a desert, except that you can't see the desert because it is not a thing.
>
> And this is why I like timetables because they make sure you don't get lost in time. (p. 195)

Occupations are what we do with our time. They provide a structure and sureness in the void of time, as the character of Christopher describes in his hatred of unorganised time. But time also provides us with a conundrum; it is essentially empty and therefore potentially infinite, and yet we can measure time though our own body's growth and decay – a very finite experience of reality. The existential analysts (Frankl and Yalom, as discussed in Hasselkus, 1997) use the nature of time to comment on the existential anxiety that each person must face. The most fundamental question is: if I am to die, if I am essentially alone (no other person like me) and if everything I do carries the ultimate responsibility of choice, then why am I here?

One of the founders of the profession of occupational therapy, Meyer (1977, originally published in 1922) wrote: 'Man learns to organize time and he does it in terms of *doing* things' (p. 642).

That each person has the capacity to organise time is a core belief in the profession, such that each person's use of time is considered unique and carries a mixture of personal meaning, cultural significance and social sanction. In an occupational therapy analysis, a patient's inner world might be explored by trying to understand what they do with their time. Activity is an expression of our connection to the world and provides us with our sense of personal integrity and belonging. Understanding what we do in the space and place of time is at the heart of the profession's endeavour.

Much of the profession's recent discourse has been focused on restrictions placed on the participation of individuals, groups or societies in occupations (Townsend, 1997; Wilcock, 1998a). Our attention is drawn to the social model of disability, which proposes that individuals are excluded from participation in many activities by society's attitude towards difference and/or disability. These issues are important and well argued by these authors, who call our attention to the need to take action on issues of 'occupational injustice' (Whiteford, 1997).

The narrative accounts of individuals who have been imprisoned and held in solitary confinement for periods of time (Sachs, 1990; Keenan, 1992) demonstrate the value of activity as a way of establishing a sense of personhood through routines which occupy time. For example, Sachs described his daily routine in prison, which included polishing a plastic water jug (one of the few objects in his prison cell) with toilet paper.

> My need for activity is desperate, but there must be some element of usefulness in what I do. If the work is completely senseless, I feel even more demoralized at its completion than if I had done nothing at all. I put the jug on the floor near the door, and start to get my clothing ready for exercise time. The procedure is similar. Each item – the sandshoes, the shorts the vest – is dealt with separately and meticulously. From the tiniest bit of work, the sort of thing one does normally and casually and without thinking, I construct a methodical and conscious labor.
>
> (Sachs, 1990, p. 55)

Harrowing accounts of the effects of occupational deprivation have given therapists a renewed interest in issues of inclusion, choice and empowerment that have taken many beyond their individual work with clients and into larger political and social arenas (Townsend, 1997; Whiteford, 1997; Wilcock, 1998a). I have welcomed this understanding of the wider realms of occupational engagement but am concerned that the language of empowerment may neglect the shadow side of disability, dependency and care.

Hoggett (2000) warned us that the pursuit of rights for individuals may blind us to understanding the inner conflicts that exist in each of us, which are not mitigated or removed in the rhetoric of empowerment. He brought to our notice the tension between the 'commitment to individual liberty . . . [and] . . . an equally passionate commitment to an ethic of care' (p. 174). The need, in some clients, for complete dependency and their inability to embrace or consider change must be seen as part of the ethics of care. The capacity to care brings with it the responsibility of concern for those individuals who may choose to hurt others or harm themselves – unconscious urges acknowledged in psychoanalytic work but frequently denied in the rhetoric of empowerment. Hoggett highlighted his concern with the potential loss of an ethic of care in health services.

> People may wish to make choices that are harmful to themselves. Joan Riviere (1936), in a powerful description of suicide, reflects on the feelings of despair and worthlessness that accompany acute depression. She illustrates how some individuals become gripped by the idea that everything they touch turns bad, they are so convinced of the actuality of their own overwhelming destructiveness that they choose death in a desperate attempt to protect those that they love and care for from themselves. This is the most extreme example of self-harm, but at what point does passionate commitment to individual liberty give way to an equally passionate commitment to an ethic of care?
>
> (Hoggett, 2000, p. 174)

My concern with recent trends in the discourse of empowerment is the potential neglect of the difficult and emotionally highly charged field of care for the individual patient, whose occupational choices may be an indication of their inner distress. I have wondered if the stirring words of emancipation and achievement are used to avoid thinking (and feeling) about the possible experiences of fear, envy, humiliation or shame of being dependent.

The choices an individual makes about how to use his time can provide us with a rich tapestry of potential meaning about his life and inner world. But activity can also be used as a defence against the difficulty of being in a place without a clear and purposeful structure, that is, our unconscious minds.

The psychoanalyst and artist, Marion Milner (1900–1998) found that it was not until she delved into her inner mind, with all its contradictions of envy, 'murderous rage and fear of retribution', that she was able to contact her 'still small voice – an alive and intuitive part, which seemed to express her real, deep needs beneath the noisy clamoring of her will and social norms' (Karph, 1999, p. iix). This process was not easy, and she became aware of 'her fear of engulfment and annihilation. But the rewards were abundant' (Karph, 1999, p. ix). These rewards may well be the capacity for creativity and reparation.

Occupations as creative expression and reparative representation

A few years ago I was listening to the author Philip Pullman being interviewed on the BBC Radio 4 programme, *Desert Island Discs* (6 October 2002). I was intrigued by his answer to the interviewer's question: 'Have you always wanted to be a writer?' He replied: 'No, I wouldn't say that I have always wanted to *be* a writer, but I have always *wanted to write.*'

It seemed to me that this is one of the indications of the creative process, that the person has a desire to enact a certain process that results in a substantial piece of work, such as a book, painting or political activity. Although I have been critical of occupations that may represent (for an individual) a defence against their feelings of dependence, occupations can also be a result of an emotional commitment to a relationship and represent the value of relationships with others. Milner (1996) described having to let go of wholly conscious processes in order to find a wonder in the unknown. What she referred to is the exploration of the unconscious as a source of creativity and pleasure.

Segal (1986), a Kleinian analyst, wrote that one source of creativity is the capacity of an individual to feel guilt and a sense of responsibility towards others. This, in part, is a result of the individual being able to enter 'the depressive position' (p. 69), which is highlighted by an appreciation that their primary object (usually the mother) is both a source of pleasure and of frustration. In other words, the person is a *whole object* and therefore someone (an object) whom the baby can both love and hate in equal measures. The realisation that the mother is both the person who feeds the baby (that is, the good mother/breast) and the person who frustrates the baby by not responding immediately to a cry for food or comfort (that is, the bad mother/breast) puts the child in touch with his guilt about having bad feelings towards the mother and the possibility that he could harm her.

> In the depressive position, anxieties spring from ambivalence, and the child's main anxiety is that his own destructive impulses have destroyed, or will destroy, the object that he loves and totally depends on.
>
> (Segal, 1988, p. 69)

This description does not only belong to the child's realisation that the person he loves and depends on is also the person with whom he is angry, or towards whom he feels hateful, it can be seen in many adult relationships. Craib (1994) referred to this when he spoke about the 'dreadful complexity' (p. vi) of relationships that are often charged with ambivalence. A person, in accepting that she can love and hate the same person, realises that she can potentially harm and may have hurt (damaged) her loved other. At this point, the desire for reparation is most strongly felt, and this can lead to actions which result in creative endeavours such as works of art or maybe an action towards the restoration or promotion of social justice.

> The reparative drives bring about a further step in integration. Love is brought more sharply into conflict with hate, and it is active in both controlling

destructiveness and in repairing and restoring damage done. It is the wish and capacity for restoration of the good object, internal and external, that is the basis for the ego's capacity to maintain love and relationships through conflicts and difficulties. It is also the basis for creative activities, which are rooted in the infant's wish to restore and recreate his lost happiness, his lost internal objects and the harmony of his internal world.

(Segal, 1988, p. 92)

Craib (1994) used the Kleinian concept of the depressive position and its concomitant defence of a reparative drive in a commonsense way that speaks to the reader of everyday concerns. He wrote about the difficulty people have in managing the ambivalence (love and hate) that they feel in any loving relationship, and how this ability to manage our feelings creates an inner morality

concerning our ability to maintain and re-establish good inner objects in the face of anxiety and rage . . . In practical terms, it seems to me to involve holding onto our ability to put the other's interests before our own . . .

(Segal, 1988, p. 173).

My interest in occupations is related to the opportunities they present for us to be creative, and to the possibility that our desire to engage in them may come from this need to make reparation. Segal (1988) said that the artist is 'primarily concerned with their restoration of his objects' (p. 214) and that the creative process is both the creation of the object and the making amends for past 'enormities'. She cited the author, Proust, who said:

. . . a book, like memory, is 'a vast graveyard where on most of the tombstones one can no longer read the faded names.' To him writing a book is bringing this lost world of loved objects back to life: 'I had to recapture from the shade that which I had felt, to re-convert it into its psychic equivalent, but the way to do it, the only way I could see, what was it but to create a work of art'.

(Segal, 1986, p. 214)

The potential of the unconscious mind and the processes that occur which result in action in the form of occupation may be worthy of further thought by occupational therapists. Collins (2001) encouraged therapists to explore the edge between the known and unknown. Although he did not call this edge the interface between the conscious and unconscious, he was critical of the way we have used consciousness to restrict our capacity to change.

The whole question of human adaptation not only rests on whether one has the physical, psychological, spiritual, social, economic or practice resources and skills to meet change, but must also reflect the ways in which individuals can be creative or sufficiently empowered to consider a range of options for action . . . Human occupation is concerned with many facets of life and inevitably involves meeting edges, struggles, conflicts and disappointments.

(Collins, 2001, p. 27)

Lawrence (2003) wrote about the 'positive aspects of the unconscious, which is the source of thinking and creativity' (p. 621). He described the unconscious as the source of mankind's wisdom – we only know it through its symbolic representations, one of which is our dreams. Collins (2004) encouraged therapists to listen to their clients' dreams as a way of anticipating and encouraging change, but he did not propose a fuller involvement in a psychoanalytic discourse within the profession. However, this article provides a window into other ways of seeing: perhaps if we could look at our own dreams about our work as well as those of our clients we would be embarking on a voyage of discovery that has been prohibited in the recent emphasis in occupational therapy on evidence-based practice and measurable outcomes.

Pullman (1995), in his children's book, *Northern Lights*, introduced to the story a wondrous instrument, the alethiometer, which when used correctly 'tells the truth' (p. 127). Its purpose is to answer the questions of the reader and thereby provide guidance on the possible consequences of action. It is depicted as a circular object (like a compass) with a needle that moves in response to the focused thought or inner (unspoken) question of the reader. The needle rests momentarily on a certain pattern of symbols arranged around the perimeter of the face. To understand the meaning of the answer, the reader must allow a loss of focus on the reality of the moment and see beneath the surface representation of the symbol to the possible underlying meanings. Each symbol carries many potential meanings (for example, the sun may symbolise day, authority, truth, kingship, and so on) and these meanings can only be understood in relation to the other identified symbols and the intention of the enquiry.

The complex process of reading the alethiometer, described in the book, may be a way we could look at the meaning of an occupation for our patients. We would start with the purpose of the question and the pointer, which moves from symbol to symbol, could identify potential meanings within the person's social, political, cultural and unconscious life, and these meanings could only be understood in relation to each other.

The use of activities in our work with clients is a valued and distinguishing aspect of our work as occupational therapists. Understanding the possible meaning of an activity for someone can deepen the relationship we establish with a patient, as well as providing us with a therapeutic agent of change. Fidler and Fidler (1978, p. 306) wrote: '. . . when an activity relates both realistically and symbolically to an individual's needs and personal characteristics it is an agent for learning and growth'.

In ending this section I wanted to use an example of an activity which provided a shift in a young client's life so that she could develop into a less introverted adult and begin her first love relationship (Box 4.1).

Box 4.1

In 1992, a 17-year-old woman, Clara, was referred to an anxiety management group which I ran in an outpatient mental health clinic. Since leaving school, the previous year, she had begun to experience panic attacks and found it more and more difficult to leave her parental home. She said she wanted to get a job and have a life outside of her home, but she was often filled with fear about what might happen to herself or her family if she went away.

The group, which used a six-week cognitive behavioural programme, encouraged clients to bring examples of situations in their own lives to use in the role-plays and other behavioural strategies. Clara seemed to benefit from the group interaction and feedback and she described being considerably less anxious after attending all six sessions. Shortly after this, she was able to secure some employment in a clothing warehouse and she asked to see me individually to work on her self-confidence.

She told me of some of the reasons for her underlying anxieties. She was one of three children, with a much older brother and a younger sister. She described how she and her sister were very close, both in age and appearance; she said they were often mistaken for twins. When her sister was 13 years old and Clara was only 14½, her sister developed a sudden and serious kidney disease and died.

Clara said that her sister's death had been devastating for the family and she traced some of her anxiety symptoms back to that time. Clara's description of her family's grief and her own sense of loss made me think that time (and therefore development) in her life had come to a standstill since her sister's death. I suggested that Clara might want to write a letter to her sister as if she were alive today, but living in another place. I cannot say why I suggested a letter, perhaps because writing to friends seemed in keeping with what teenagers did then – not unlike the use of mobile phone texting or emailing nowadays. Clara was intrigued by the idea and said she would try it out.

The following week Clara brought a long letter she had written to her sister. Many of the details have been lost to my memory, and she kept it so I could not refer to it later, but I do remember the following. Clara told her sister how much she missed her and would still like to talk to her, but the surprise in the letter was how much Clara resented her for her death. Clara said her sister had become the idealized daughter – the daughter whose picture was kept on the mantelpiece, who could be dusted and remembered as perfect and who never got older or disappointed her parents. Clara felt the burden of constantly comparing herself to this perfect daughter.

Following the discovery of her resentment towards this idealised image of her sister, Clara began to change. She was able to recognise that her sister had been frozen in time but that she (Clara) needed to move on and in reality would be (and needed to be) different from her. Over the next three months Clara's confidence increased in her personal relationships and she described having fun with the people that she worked with. She began to dress differently, wearing the more modern jeans and t-shirts of her peer group and not the younger style of dress she had previously chosen. She also indicated there was a young man at work she liked and she subsequently began a relationship with him. It was at that point we ended the therapy as she no longer had any panic attacks and was able to leave her home to meet up with friends with few anxiety symptoms.

Creek (1997a) wrote that occupational therapists 'aim to make small but significant changes in the lives of their clients in order to help the clients to develop a sense of being able to manage better' (p. 51). Although I did not see Clara again and do not know if she continued to be free of the symptoms that initially drove her to seek help, I do think that the letter she wrote released her anger, envy and pain at the loss of her sister. This allowed her to move forward in her own life, now having a separate identity from that of her sister and perhaps being more able to learn from the inevitable experiences and disappointments of her adult life.

Occupational therapy on the couch

This last section is an attempt to consolidate some of my thoughts on occupational therapy with respect to the work of the psychoanalytically orientated organisational consultants who have examined the culture of institutions and/or professional groups. They have attempted to understand how institutions both conceive of their tasks and manage their work loads by considering the conscious and unconscious mechanisms that can impact on the individual worker and the context of care. The work of these consultants helps me to understand why some institutions, which were created to provide care and rehabilitation for vulnerable individuals, often seem to do quite the opposite (Menzies Lyth, 1988; Miller, 1993; Obholzer and Roberts, 1994; Trist and Murray, 1990) (Box 4.2).

Box 4.2

In 1993, a friend of mine was involved in a serious car accident and sustained an incomplete lesion to his C5 cerebral vertebra, leaving him initially paralysed from his shoulder girdle (with some movement in his upper arm) down to his feet. During his period of recovery I visited him several times, in the specialist spinal rehabilitation hospital, and was dismayed and concerned to observe several aspects of uncaring towards not only him but also other patients whose mobility was severely restricted through spinal injury.

The hospital was built in a series of single-storey wards that sprawled out over a large area and were linked by a series of concrete pathways. These pathways were created to facilitate wheelchair-bound patients' mobility from ward to rehabilitation centres; however, they showed signs of severe neglect. Many of the grass verges had grown over or through the concrete, making many of the paths impassible to any person using a wheelchair. This in effect forced patients using wheelchairs onto the narrow roads, whose one-way traffic system often left clients vulnerable to the build-up of hospital and public transport.

It seemed to me that a hospital whose stated aim was the rehabilitation of patients with spinal cord injuries was providing a significant obstacle to this stated aim by neglecting (or denying) that the environment of care did not allow for the free movement of people using wheelchairs. There may have been many conscious reasons (such as budget cuts) why the grass had not been attended to but I wondered if the neglect of the environment had to do with an institution that unconsciously denied the extent of disability in the clients. Many of the clients who depended on wheelchairs or trolleys for some mobility and independence of movement could no longer negotiate the paths without assistance. It was as if the institution had itself become paralysed and unable to respond to the needs of its clients.

The notion of an organisational culture that is partially created and influenced by unconscious anxieties evoked by the nature of the work was highlighted in a study undertaken by Menzies Lyth (1988) with nursing staff. She said that the culture of an institution, which can inform the policy and procedures of that institution and influence its primary task, may be established as a defence against the primitive unconscious anxieties that arise from the workers' direct contact with clients. Occupational therapists may be employing a similar mechanism of a social/professional defence against intimate contact with clients who, by virtue of trauma, illness or hereditary disorder, are temporarily or permanently dependent on heath care and often viewed by society as disabled.

A significant dream

I have been an occupational therapist since 1979. I began training after my final year at school and have not done any other professional work. Most of my endeavours with clients have had a focus on activities that would encourage and/or return them to health. I held a strong belief in the efficacy of doing as a way of restoring well-being and, in many respects, this belief echoed my personal life, which involved many outdoor activities and social engagements.

In 1996, following a sabbatical in the UK where I was introduced to the work of Menzies Lyth (1988) through a course undertaken at the Institute of Group Analysis, I had the following dream (Box 4.3). It unsettled me greatly because it questioned the assumptions I had made about my professional role and identity. Although the dream clearly indicated that I needed to pay attention to my own psychic soul, it is its reference to the professional work I had undertaken over the last 20 years that made me think differently about the professional discourse of occupational therapy.

Box 4.3

In the dream I had a deep wound on my lower leg, and I went to a doctor to ask for his help. He said that the wound was serious and that I would have to have my leg amputated. I said that if that were the case I would do it myself. I went home and planned to cut off my own leg with my grandfather's sword (a family heirloom that had always been part of my life). However I did not have the courage to do it and so I returned to the doctor and asked if there was any other way of saving my leg. He asked a female colleague to see me and after her consultation she said that it was good news, my leg did not have to be cut off, but that it would take a long time to heal. While I was relieved at the news, I felt guilty because I thought that I was an occupational therapist and, although I had encouraged people who had undergone an amputation to walk again with an artificial limb, I did not want one.

Since that time I have become aware of the overly optimistic discourse used by occupational therapists when working with or writing about clients. It seems to me that the pain of illness and the reality of social exclusion for those who have profound disabilities are denied by a professional group who see it as their job to encourage, equip or enable clients to engage again in their lives. In a recent research project, I suggested that this positive view is paramount to a dismissal of clients' real experience and represents the profession's need to maintain a comfortable distance from the very personal pain that clients bring into treatment situations.

In the mid-1990s, there was a series of jokes which began: 'How many xxxx's does it take to change a light bulb?' This recipe was applied to occupational therapists and so the joke became: 'How many OTs does it take to change a light bulb?' The answer was: 'Only one, but they don't change the light bulb, they teach you how to cope in the dark.' In this simple joke lies the inherent discomfort in a coping response to the world of darkness. Some people may not want to cope with the dark because coping may require of them to deny that there is any dark at all (Nicholls, 2003).

The culture of an institution

Menzies Lyth (1988) undertook a study at a large teaching hospital to examine the problem, at that time, of student nurse training and retention. Her work used a psychoanalytic perspective on the work situation. She described nurses' work as having to confront situations that are extraordinary and distressing and may also resemble early unconscious anxiety.

> Nurses face the reality of suffering and death as few lay people do. Their work involves carrying out tasks which by ordinary standards are distasteful, disgusting and frightening. Intimate physical contact with patients arouses libidinal and erotic wishes that may be difficult to control. The work arouses strong feelings: pity, compassion and love; guilt and anxiety; hatred and resentment of the patients who arouse those feelings; envy of the care they receive.
>
> (Menzies Lyth, in Trist and Murray, 1990, p. 440)

In order for nurses to undertake these tasks on behalf of patients and their relatives, Menzies Lyth suggested that they need to develop a professional repertoire of practices and procedures designed to protect them from excessive personal anxiety and enable them to undertake their caring role. However, her observations attested to the fact that many of these procedures do not serve that function and seem to add additional and excessive anxiety to the nursing situation. It was with these observations that Menzies Lyth drew our attention to the unconscious aspect of work and the role of institutional culture.

Menzies Lyth (1990) drew a parallel between the nursing tasks and 'the phantasy situation that exists in every individual at the deepest and most primitive level of the mind' (p. 440). She said that, because the objective features of the actual task so closely represent the symbolic fantasy of destruction and decay in the person's inner world, the nurse is both exposed to excessive anxiety and unable to master it. It is the symbolic equation of real events with imagined ones that threatens the nurse's psychic world most profoundly. Against this threat of overwhelming anxiety, nurses construct a social/professional defence, and this defence becomes encoded into the culture and task performance of nursing, influencing how and where work is done:

> the culture, structure and mode of functioning are determined by the psychological needs of the members . . . A social defense system develops over time through collusive interaction and agreement, often unconscious, between members of the organization as to what form it will take. The socially structured defense mechanisms then tend to become an aspect of external reality with which new and old members of the institution must come to terms.
> (Menzies Lyth, in Trist and Murray, 1990, p. 443)

The socially constructed defence which operates in professional groups or work situations is an unconscious mechanism and can be seen to be operating only by examining work procedures and processes and by questioning their underlying assumptions. In doing this, Menzies Lyth was able to analyse the procedures undertaken in the hospital both as defending nurses from anxiety and preventing them from progressing beyond it. She identified various practices that in theory were espoused as poor nursing care but in practice were commonplace, for example, splitting the nurse from patient, objectifying patients into conditions and ritualising the performance of tasks to avoid feeling emotional responsibility for the patient.

Menzies Lyth placed the relationship between client and health worker, with its concomitant unconscious anxiety, as the primary influence on professional and institutional culture. Although Menzies Lyth's study (undertaken in the 1960s) has been used to alert nurses to ways in which their work can be subverted through lack of attention to the relationship with their clients and its concomitant anxiety, recent authors do not think that much has changed in the nursing culture.

Fabricius (1991) said that although there have been significant changes in the professional status of nurses, they are still exposed to the raw emotion of client projections in the close daily encounters that are part of their caring work. She said that it is 'the sheer quantity, as well as force, of the projections that are thrust on them that are too much for any ordinary human . . .' (p. 103). This makes it impossible for nurses to work through the emotional impact of their work. Because of this 'sheer quantity', she maintained that nurses continue to employ a socially structured (professional) defence mechanism that curtails contact with patients and denies the emotional impact of their work that Menzies Lyth originally identified.

Fabricius (1999), in a later paper, said that 'low self esteem' (p. 203) in nursing is caused by its own members and not by political or social pressures from outside the profession. She said that nurses devalue themselves and thereby each other. She linked this with the devaluing of the original nursing role, that of a mother suckling her baby. She encouraged nurses to resume their psychological care of patients as the real task of nursing and not overvalue the technical skills and academic knowledge that nurses seem to be pursuing for internal validation and professional recognition. Nurses have chosen to perform a certain kind of work, perhaps because of deeply held beliefs and/or unconscious needs for reparation, and they should be supported in their endeavours by structures that allow for the fulfilment of this need.

Occupational therapy as a defence against dependence and disability

Occupational therapy as a profession has not had the same psychoanalytic scrutiny that the professions of nursing, medicine and social work have undergone in recent literature (Foster and Roberts, 1998; Obholzer and Roberts, 1994). I have often wondered if we have escaped the serious attention of psychodynamic authors because we lack the physical presence and drama that seem to be afforded the professions that are featured on British television programmes such as *Holby City* and *Casualty*. If we were to examine the culture of our profession and its assumptions about health, the value of independence and activity, would we discover that there are unconscious anxieties that affect our relationships with patients, and that we have resorted to the use of activities as a defence against these anxieties?

Finlay (1998), writing about the value of reflexivity in her research into the life worlds of occupational therapists, looked at her 'unconscious responses' (p. 453) to the clients she observed and the transference and countertransference she experienced with the occupational therapist she interviewed. She described how, when observing a therapist treat a patient who was dying of lung cancer, she 'could not stop herself from getting involved' (p. 454). She reflected on her difficulty with maintaining an observer role and linked it to the therapist's need to do things for the patient.

> When I reflected on my behaviour, I understood that it was due to my active need to be involved, to do something. I also recognized my own sensitivity as an asthmatic, witnessing someone with breathing problems dying of lung disease. Once I recognized this, I could then see that the occupational therapist was experiencing similar identifications with some of her other patients. Previously I had interpreted the therapist as being involved with fairly superficial,

irrelevant tasks. Now I could see that these tasks had a meaning for her – they were as much for her as for the patient.

(Finlay, 1998, p. 454)

Understanding the value and meaning of occupation and incorporating its use in treatment are core tenets of the profession. The word is, after all, in our professional title. Activities (in all their forms and complexity) have been used with clients to achieve aims as diverse as increasing muscle strength, building self-esteem or learning to cope with a diminishing memory. Some of the activities used with clients have been criticised as being reductionist and lacking in personal and cultural relevance, such as the wire twisting machine that may have increased range of shoulder movement but had little personal meaning in the client's life (Nicholls, 1992). As part of the evolution of the profession, there have been changes in the activities that are used in therapy and how they are used (Creek, 1997b; Mattingly, 1998; Serrett, 1985). There is also more sensitivity towards what has meaning for the client, but the concern in my dream remains. Are we, by using games and activities, teaching patients to cope but, with our emphasis on being busy, denying them an opportunity to heal (Box 4.4)?

Box 4.4

In 1992, while working in an outpatient community mental health team, I was asked to help a middle-aged man who had become deeply depressed following some significant losses in his life: an intimate relationship, his work and, linked to these, his accommodation. This was his first contact with mental health services and his history demonstrated that he had been successful in many areas of his life prior to this mid-life breakdown, indicating that with some support and skill training he might readily improve. Nothing prepared me for the therapeutic journey this man and I were to embark on over the next year.

He saw me on a weekly basis and, although I tried every strategy I knew as an occupational therapist to encourage him to seek new avenues of work, or re-engage in social pastimes, he became more depressed and eventually significantly suicidal. At the point when I was going to refer him back to the acute services for a possible admission, he began to tell me the story of his life. I did not always feel I was equipped or trained to respond to the extent of his revelations, which included his having been repeatedly sexually abused by a parent from the age of 8 to 15 years of age. I was reluctant to refer him on as he said he had never told this to anyone before, and he might view a ▶

referral to another professional as a rejection. He may have felt that his revelations could have damaged or contaminated his relationship with me and so, with the support of my supervisor, I saw the patient each week and he spoke about himself.

The patient made progress in the year-long period of his occupational therapy but I still cannot think of one thing I **did** to help him. During the latter half of his treatment he was able to engage in training for a new career, leading to new employment, and he joined a social group based on a previous interest of his.

When we saw each other for the last time, I asked what had helped him the most. It was a genuine question, as I was still unsure what had happened to help him make a recovery. He said what had helped him was that I could listen to how awful he felt week by week, when he did not tell, and had never told, anyone else. He said that being able to 'say it like it was' week by week gave him the courage to keep going and, after a time, begin to try again with aspects of his life, such as his work and meeting people.

Recent occupational therapy literature, in an attempt to reclaim our past traditions and philosophies, has emphasised both the value of doing occupations with clients and the need for a positive view of ourselves (Mayers, 2000; Wilcock, 2002). While carrying out a study of professional identity (Nicholls, 2003), I was struck by the number of references therapists made to their positive view of their work with clients: words describing pain, confusion and disillusionment were entirely absent from their conversation.

Occupational therapy literature is full of positive statements about the role and value of occupational therapy, only recently occupational therapists were told that to be positive was a 'professional imperative' (Bannigan, 2002, p. 397). One need only look at the title of the forthcoming conference of occupational therapists who work in mental health (AOTMH), 'Enable, Equip and Empower,' to realize that occupational therapists have used this discourse of positive upbeat emancipation as a given in nearly all professional contexts. What seems to have been lost (or avoided) is that experiences with clients can be painful and unrewarding, and that we as a professional group are sometimes not sure of who we are, or why we do what we do, and if we have made a difference to our clients.

(Nicholls, 2003, p. 34)

Roberts (1994), in writing about a consultation she had done in a long-term care institution, suggested that occupational therapists employ a socially structured defence in their work with older adults. She used a term that was initially coined by Miller and Gwynne (cited in Roberts, 1994), *the horticultural model of care*. This, she said, means that occupational therapists believe that all patients want to grow, do more and become independent of the care that is part of the residential institution. She said that there is 'excessive praise for minor achievements' with an accompanying 'denial of disabilities' (p. 80). In the end, the patients are sure to disappoint the therapists as they cannot maintain this level of independence.

> A good inmate here is one happy, fulfilled, active and independent. Eventually, of course nearly all of them fail.
>
> (Roberts, in Obholzer and Roberts, 1994, p. 80)

Another example of the denial of disability is those teachers and physiotherapists at a school for profoundly disabled children who encourage the children's ambitions to be train drivers or bus conductors (Obholzer and Roberts, 1994). Although occupational therapists were not mentioned as promoting the children's employment aspirations, I think this stands as an example of the defence system that therapists employ to protect themselves from the full force of the anguish of a profound disability. There is a temptation to deny the painful reality of the social exclusion that will face these children when they leave the safe confines of a school that is specially adapted for their needs.

Occupational therapists tend to see the main goal of their work as promoting independence (Mayers, 2000; Reilly, 1985). Alongside a belief in the individual's desire for self-efficacy and independence there is a clear distinction between the professional role and the client's experience. Therapists did not see themselves, in my study (2003) or in the recent literature, as requiring the help they so readily offer to their patients. This denial of the need for dependency in others or oneself could be a symptom of the profession's unconscious defense against vulnerability and thereby affect its professional role in health care. Hoggett (2000) drew our attention to the hatred of dependency that has been reinforced in modern cultural assumptions about interdependence.

> Vulnerability and dependence are not just things which are imminent, i.e. potentially waiting round the corner for us. These things are also immanent, i.e. dwelling within each of us. Inside each of us there is a small child which is open to wonder and yet so easily hurt. Inside each of us there is a drifter and nomad, a failure, a non-survivor and all the persons that the passive internal voice can assume. A good society would be one which could provide a place for such selves to be, without always seeking to empower them or thrust cures

upon them. Sometimes people just want to rest and be taken care of, sometimes people just want to drift along without having to think too much.

(Hoggett, 2000, p. 169)

In my dream I decided to cut off my own leg, not because I was strong and brave but because I was ashamed of needing help from another. When (in the dream) I realised I did not have to live an adapted life (with an artificial leg), I was ashamed that I had expected so many of my clients to enact that very denial of a wound that may require a good deal of time to heal.

In an earlier section, I discussed the Kleinian theory of the unconscious mechanisms that are employed by individuals to cope with the realization of their dependence on, and thereby the possibility of their damaging, others. These defences fall under two headings, the manic defence and the reparative defence. I wondered if the doing part of occupational therapy is at times a manic defence, as if the client should not (and thereby does not) experience the painfulness of social exclusion. Many of our clients do not have sudden remissions or a return to a healthy functioning, and there may be no possibility of the work, social networks or leisure pursuits that occupational therapists so enthusiastically promote. Reparative defences, which acknowledge the responsibility that we have for our actions, allow the individual to mature, but it is a 'slow process and it takes a long time for the ego to acquire sufficient strength to feel confident in its reparative capacities' (Segal, 1988, p. 2) (Box 4.5).

Box 4.5

At a recent conference for occupational therapists who work in mental health (2003) a keynote speaker discussed her experience of mental illness. In a very moving and candid manner, she spoke of her psychotic illness and showed a video taken of her during her illness. In the video she was engaged in doing art work and her commentary described the experience of her voices, what they said to her and how they affected her difficulty in trusting the help she was given.

The speaker said she is an occupational therapist and works with clients who have mental health concerns. She wanted to share with the audience some of her insights into the process of illness and recovery. When there was an opportunity for questions, I asked what had helped her to heal and what had helped her to cope. She replied that the skills groups (mainly run by occupational therapists) helped her to cope again, but she thought her healing had been in the periods she had in art therapy, where she could express her madness.

I wonder if we, as a profession, have lost too many of the ideas that Fidler and Fidler (1963) explored when they described the use of creative activities with clients to enhance the client's communication process. Banks and Blair (1997), in writing about the use of activities in a group with older clients, said that activities such as art and music 'provide an alternative to verbal means of expression of the unconscious through the process of the activity through the end product' (p. 89). Perhaps in neglecting the importance of the unconscious we have lost a range and depth of creative activities that may allow clients to express and experience themselves in a way that allows for insight, emotional expression and healing. These aspects of work within the creative process, that can promote healing, are essentially reparative activities, stemming from the unconscious need to make sense of the world and express the self.

In conclusion

I want to return to a conclusion I came to in my study of the professional identity of occupational therapists working in multidisciplinary teams. The occupational therapists I interviewed had the capacity and eloquence to give a coherent account of their work with clients and of their professional role. The overly optimistic emphasis they gave to their work may have been in response to the research inquiry process, or an indication of a defence against the years of the profession's lowly position in the hierarchy of health care (Serrett, 1985). However, the imperative call for therapists to maintain this optimism and positive attitude may have prevented a deeper exploration and thereby an understanding of a valuable professional group.

> Perhaps what the profession needs are more opportunities to articulate their understanding of their work with clients. But it may not only be opportunity that occupational therapists require, but other words (and meanings) in their language. The dispossession of psychoanalytic thinking in the profession has been a particularly painful loss for the researcher. The analytic discourse gives a richness of description and understanding to people's life pain and dramas that seemed to have been lost in the language of clearly stated goals and outcomes that have been part of the occupational therapy literature today.
>
> (Nicholls, 2003)

Psychoanalysis, with its theories of the unconscious, libidinal drives and the importance of object relationships, gives us a powerful and varied language to express and explore the nature of what it is to be human. It allows for contradiction and uncertainty and thereby for new knowledge to emerge. Perhaps occupational therapists may be encouraged to (re-)engage in a psychoanalytic discourse in their work by discovering this way of working for themselves through the use of a reflexive clinical reasoning (that is, an examination of their unconscious responses to patients) within a containing supervisory relationship, as suggested by Daniel and Blair (2002a, b).

The language of psychoanalysis can also provide us with a way of understanding ourselves, the relationships we establish and the society in which we live. Archbishop Desmond Tutu, when asked for his opinion on the war in Iraq and the Palestinian–Israeli conflict, used the African word 'Ubuntu', which means that a person is only a person through his relationships with other people. The Archbishop used this word to describe the responsibility we all carry towards each other. This helped me to understand the following passage again and for the first time.

> . . . the straightforward rejection of the insights of psychotherapy does not help, because it denies one of the few areas where a separation from the system can be achieved: the complex internality of the individual, comprehension of which can enable him or her to take a critical and analytic distance from what is happening, and enable the formation of relationships based less on the illusion of common identity than on the reality of individual separation, difference and dependence. But this achievement means recognition of the real internal pain of fragmentation, of internal conflicts and of our manifold limitations. This, perhaps, is the most important message of psychoanalysis.
>
> (Craib, 1994, p. 189)

What I think he is saying is that psychoanalysis gives us an opportunity to think about ourselves and our capacity to feel concern for others, and a critical ability to see through rhetoric and cultural assumptions about what is right or good for oneself or others. It is this ability to think about our feelings and experiences that emancipates us and allows us to love the other as a separate and important part of our lives.

References

Banks, E.J. and Blair, S.E.E. (1997) The contribution of occupational therapy within the context of the psychodynamic approach for older clients who have mental health problems. *Health Care in Later Life*, **2**(2), 85–92.

Bannigan, K. (2002) A positive attitude is a professional imperative. *British Journal of Occupational Therapy*, **6**(9), 397.

Bateman, A. and Holmes, J. (1995) *Introduction to Psychoanalysis*, Brunner-Routledge, London.

Bion, W.R. (1967) *Second Thoughts*, Karnac Books, London.

Bion, W.R. (1991) *The Long Weekend*, Karnac Books, London.

Bonington, C. (2001) *The Everest Years*, Weidenfeld & Nicolson, London.

Brown, D. and Peddar, J. (1991) *Introduction to Psychotherapy*, 2nd edn, Routledge, London.

Christiansen, C.H. (1999) Defining lives: occupation as identity: an essay on competence, coherence, and the creation of meaning. *American Journal of Occupational Therapy*, **53**(6), 547–58.

Christiansen, C. and Baum, C. (1997) *Occupational Therapy Enabling Function and Well-Being*, 2nd edn, Slack, Thorofare, NJ.

Cole, M. (1998) *Group Dynamics in Occupational Therapy*, Slack, Thorofare, NJ.

Collins, M. (2001) Who is occupied? Consciousness, self awareness and the process of human adaptation. *Journal of Occupational Science*, **8**(1), 25–32.

Collins, M. (2004) Dreaming and occupation. *British Journal of Occupational Therapy*, **67**(2), 96–8.

Craib, I. (1994) *The Importance of Disappointment*, Routledge, London.

Craib, I. (2001) *Psychoanalysis: A Critical Introduction*, Polity Press, Cambridge, UK.

Creek, J. (1997a) The truth is no longer out there. *British Journal of Occupational Therapy*, **60**(2), 50–2.

Creek, J. (1997b) *Occupational Therapy and Mental Health*, 2nd edn, Churchill Livingstone, Edinburgh.

Daniel, M. and Blair, S. (2002a) A psychodynamic approach to clinical supervision: 1. *British Journal of Therapy and Rehabilitation*, **9**(6), 237–40.

Daniel, M. and Blair, S. (2002b) A psychodynamic approach to clinical supervision: 2. *British Journal of Therapy and Rehabilitation*, **9**(7), 274–7.

De Saint-Exupery, A. (1974) *The Little Prince*, Pan Books Ltd, UK.

Fabricius, J. (1991) Running on the spot or can nursing really change? *Psychoanalytic Psychotherapy*, **5**(2), 97–108.

Fabricius, J. (1999) The crisis in nursing: reflections on the crisis. *Psychoanalytic Psychotherapy*, **13**(3), 203–6.

Fearing, V. and Clark, J. (2000) *Individuals in Context*. Slack, Thorofare, NJ.

Fidler, G. and Fidler, J. (1963) *Occupational Therapy as a Communication Process in Psychiatry*, Macmillan Publishing Co., New York.

Fidler, G. and Fidler, J. (1978) Doing and becoming: purposeful action and self-actualization. *American Journal of Occupational Therapy*, **32**(5), 305–10.

Finlay, L. (1998) Reflexivity: an essential component for all research? *British Journal of Occupational Therapy*, **61**(10), 453–6.

Foster, A. and Roberts, V.A. (1998) *Managing Mental Health in the Community*, Routledge, London.

Haddon, M. (2003) *The Curious Incident of the Dog in the Night-Time*, Jonathan Cape, London.

Hagedorn, R. (1992) *Occupational Therapy: Foundations for Practice*, Churchill Livingstone, Edinburgh.

Hasselkus, B.R. (1997) Meaning and occupation, in *Occupational Therapy: Enabling Function and Well-Being*, 2nd edn (C. Christiansen and C. Baum), Slack, Thorofare, NJ.

Hasselkus, B.R. (2002) *The Meaning of Everyday Occupation*, Slack, Thorofare, NJ.

Hoggett, P. (2000) Hatred of dependency, in *Emotional Life and the Politics of Welfare*, Macmillan, Basingstoke, UK.

Karpf, A. (1999) Marion Milner, Journey to the Centre of the Mind, in *A Life of One's Own* (M. Milner), Virago, London.

Keenan, B. (1992) *An Evil Cradling*, Hutchinson, London.

Keilhofner, G. (1995) *A Model of Human Occupation: Theory and Application*, Williams and Wilkins, Baltimore.

Kielhofner, G. and Burke, J. (1977) Occupational therapy after 60 years: an account of changing identity and knowledge. *American Journal of Occupational Therapy*, **31**(10), 675–89.

Krakauer, J. (1997) *Into Thin Air: A Personal Account of the Mount Everest Disaster*, Macmillan, Basingstoke, UK.

Lawrence, W.G. (2003) Social dreaming as sustained thinking. *Human Relations*, **56**(5), 609–24.

Mattingly, C. (1998) *Healing Dramas and Clinical Plots: The Narrative Structure of Experience*, Cambridge University Press, Cambridge, UK.

Mayers, C.A. (2000) The Casson Memorial Lecture 2000: Reflect on the past to shape the future. *British Journal of Occupational Therapy*, **63**(8), 358–66.

Menzies Lyth, I. (1988) *Containing Anxiety in Institutions*, Free Association Books, London.

Menzies Lyth, I. (1990) Social systems as a defense against anxiety, in *The Social Engagement of Social Science* (E. Trist and H. Murray), Free Association Books, London.

Meyer, A. (1977) The philosophy of occupation therapy. *American Journal of Occupational Therapy*, **31**(10), 639–42 (originally published in 1922).

Miller, E. (1993) *From Dependency to Autonomy*, Free Association Books, London.

Milner, M. (1996) *The Suppressed Madness of Sane Men*, Routledge, London.

Milner, M. (1999) *A Life of One's Own*, Virago, London.

Nicholls, L. (1992) looking behind to get ahead: occupational therapy in perspective, in *Van den Ende Memorial Lectures*, University of Cape Town, South Africa.

Nicholls, L. (2003) Factors in mental health multidisciplinary teamwork that impact on the professional identity of occupational therapists. Unpublished research project, Department of Heath and Social Care, Brunel University, London.

Obholzer, A. and Roberts, V. (eds) (1994) *The Unconscious at Work*, Routledge, London.

Pullman, P. (1998) *Northern Lights*, Scholastic Children's Books, London.

Reilly, M. (1985) Occupational therapy can be one of the Great Ideas of 20th century medicine, in *A Professional Legacy: the Eleanor Clarke Slagle Lectures 1955–1985*. (American Occupational Therapy Association) AOTA, Rockville, MD.

Roberts, V.Z. (1994) Till Death us do Part: caring and uncaring work with the elderly, in *The Unconcious @ Work* (ed. A. Obholzer and V. Roberts) Routledge, London.

Rose, D. and Douglas, E. (1999) *Regions of the Heart*, Michael Joseph, London.

Sachs, A. (1990) *The Jail Diary of Albie Sachs*, David Phillips, Cape Town, South Africa.

Segal, H. (1986) *The Work of Hanna Segal, Delusion and Artistic Creativity and Other Psychoanalytic Essays*, Free Association Books, London.

Segal, H. (1988) *Introduction to the Work of Melanie Klein*, Karnac Books, London.

Serrett, K.D. (ed.) (1985) *Philosophical and Historical Roots of Occupational Therapy*, Haworth Press, New York.

Simpson, J. (1997a) *Dark Shadows Falling*, Vintage, London.

Simpson, J. (1997b) *Touching the Void*, Vintage, London.

Townsend, E. (1997) Occupation: potential for personal and social transformation. *Journal of Occupational Science*, **4**(1), 19–26.

Townsend, E. (eds) (1997) *Enabling Occupation: An Occupational Therapy Perspective*, CAOT Publications, Ottawa.

Trist, E. and Murray, H. (1990) *The Social Engagement of Social Science*, Volume 1, Free Association Books, London.

Whiteford, G. (1997) Occupational deprivation and incarceration. *Journal of Occupational Science: Australia*, **4**(3), 126–30.

Whiteford, G., Townsend, E. and Hocking, C. (2000) Reflections and renaissance of occupation. *Canadian Journal Occupational Therapy* **67**(1), 61–9.

Wilcock, A.A. (1998a) *An Occupational Perspective of Health*, Slack, Thorofare, NJ.

Wilcock, A.A. (1998b) Reflections on doing, being and becoming. *Canadian Journal of Occupational Therapy*, **65**(5), 248–56.

Wilcock, A.A. (2001) Occupational science: the key to broadening horizons. *British Journal of Occupational Therapy*, **64**(8), 412–17.

Wilcock, A.A. (2002) A theory of the human need for occupation. *Journal of Occupational Science*, 9 (special edition), 3–9.

Yerxa, E.J. (1998) Health and the human spirit for occupation. *American Journal of Occupational Therapy*, **52**(6), 412–18.

Zemke, R. and Clark, F. (1996) *Occupational Science: The Evolving Discipline*, F.A. Davis Company, Philadelphia.

What's going on? Finding an explanation for what we do

5

Rosemary Caulton and Rayna Dickson

Introduction

It is important for a practitioner who is responsible for a professional service to be able to articulate the reasons for doing what he or she does. If one lays claim to particular wisdom and skill in relation to a particular area of human need, then knowing, showing and telling are fundamental requirements and obligations. In an educational setting, where one is preparing those who are to take up this responsibility, this obligation is paramount. So one devises and refers to understandings, theories and frameworks that have been passed on through tradition and research and that form the profession's body of knowledge. It is through this knowledge base, and by our works, that we are known. As educators at the Otago Polytechnic School of Occupational Therapy, we feel that this knowing, showing and telling is important to our professional credibility.

Occupational therapy students undergo alternating periods of academic study and fieldwork experience during their pre-registration education. The Otago Polytechnic School of Occupational Therapy has always had a commitment to community collaboration and to a strongly practical curriculum. For one of their fieldwork placements, students have the opportunity to participate in local, community-based programmes in and around Dunedin, in settings where an ongoing need for activity and community integration has been identified and a service provided to meet this need.

Stories from each placement's network of campus staff, students, practitioners and clients, as well as our own observations, tell us about the services and how they work. What we see going on across all these programmes is very similar, but how to explain it? Practitioners, rightly, focus on the services they are offering rather than on the formal articulation of what they are doing. We, as educators, however, are increasingly faced with a simple but very important need: to identify ways to articulate what students encounter in these community-based placements.

In this chapter, we draw together the understandings we have gained through practice observations in local, community-based programmes, exploration of the common usage of the word *occupation* and ongoing investigations in the literature of anthropology, labour, art and craft, as well as imaginative and professional literature. We show how all these together form a coherent body of knowledge that speaks to practice in these programmes. This body of knowledge indicates:

1. the centrality of culture in occupational practice;
2. the significance of the humanities (including imaginative literature) in understanding occupational practice; and
3. the two key roles (invisible and visible) of an occupational practitioner.

Israel Scheffler (1985) said about professions and their bodies of knowledge:

> The organisation of a practical theory is dictated, not by the aims of advancing general understanding, but by the effort to guide decision in some realm of practice. It is the practical questions of such a realm which provide the common focus for the elements of its practical theory . . . For it is the task of the professional to draw together the understandings gained by relevant disciplines, and apply them, under the guidance of an ethical ideal, to the problems of ordinary experience. (pp. 4–5)

Ideas such as this are well understood and have been spoken of in occupational therapy literature, notably by Ann Cronin Mosey, in *Configuration of a Profession* (1985). Mosey pointed out that the disciplines which are considered relevant by a profession contribute to the domain of concern, ethical code, legitimate tools and philosophical assumptions of the profession, not only in a very broad and inclusive way but in very specific and specialised areas as well. Because of this, choosing where to seek knowledge and what to look for are clearly of paramount importance.

Practice

We begin with practice because that is where the problem of explanation arose, and in relation to which all our reflection has been carried out, but it is important to remember that all of the observation, listening, discussions and reading were going on at the same time. This means that insights, information and intuitions were in a constantly symbiotic and evolving relationship.

We have collated observations of practice that have been recorded over the years (and are still current) in a selection of the student placement settings that seemed to be working well. While these observations are only very briefly outlined, we need to give sufficient detail about what was being done so that it can be seen how the explanation reflects the practice facts. It is not possible to have an explanation without there being something to explain, and we wanted to *show* that there is a necessary connection here between practice and explanation.

The settings referred to in this account are:

- a day programme for people with long-term mental health problems;
- a hospice providing a combination of inpatient, respite and day care;
- a suburban family centre providing support for mothers and babies considered to be at risk;
- a sheltered workshop for people with a mixed range of intellectual, psychiatric and physical disabilities;
- a residential programme for young men who have come through the justice system;
- a community art studio and gallery for artists who use mental health services;
- a weekly activity group for elderly men in a rest home; and
- a weekly activity group for people with acquired brain injury.

Key activities

In the apparently diverse programmes throughout Dunedin, where our students had their fieldwork experiences, people were involved in ordinary day-to-day makings and doings. Some of the programmes have a particular focus, for example the sheltered workshop and the art studio, while others function more as general activity centres. Despite this wide variation, some key activities go on in all of them.

Being part of an economic system

People are involved in the production, distribution and exchange of commodities in some shape or form. These include the direct exchange of goods and services, either among participants or between the programme and the local community, through sales tables and jumble sales. People also visit local markets and 'opportunity shops', usually for personal goods and clothing but also for materials, equipment and produce for communal activities. These activities enable participants to obtain cheaply the things they need and to raise funds for additional activities such as holidays.

Being a producer of goods and provider of services

Vegetables are grown for sale, and chutneys, cordials, jams and sweets are made for the jumble sale or monthly local markets. Greetings cards are made in the hospice and sold to raise funds. Christmas tree and firewood schemes are run, and gardening services are provided for regular customers. Voluntary work is done for the service provider, such as stuffing envelopes and removing buttons from recycled clothing. Paid employment is the primary focus of the sheltered workshop, in which typical production line work is carried out for local business and industry. Items are not only made to sell, exchange or barter but are made by the men in the residential programme for themselves or as gifts for friends and relatives.

Making things that they cannot afford to buy is particularly important for young mothers, and ideas for craft projects come from many places, such as shops or markets. These might include, for example, home-made soap, simple toys, handmade paper, cards, chocolates and basic cosmetics. The studio artists frequently use their gallery space to exhibit works for sale and reflection. Sometimes, people contribute in different ways towards the same communal project, such as making a mural to decorate an entrance or a bird pudding to feed hungry birds at the hospice.

Producing, procuring, preparing and sharing food

As might be expected whenever people come together, communal eating is part of all the programmes and is often much more than just a meal or snack. It provides a focus for people's collective attention. The production and sharing of a low-cost midday meal, with its associated menu planning and shopping, are important. At least three of the programmes tend a garden that produces food. The produce is never relied upon entirely but provides, for example, rhubarb pie for dessert or herbs for the soup for lunch.

Stopping for a coffee or smoking break and for lunch is part of the routine of workshop environments. Food is also a central focus for any special celebration. Making a cake or a special morning or afternoon tea, is a common way to celebrate an anniversary or someone's birthday or their moving on.

Food preparation always involves cleaning up afterwards, and usually involves rosters and taking turns.

General maintenance and management

This is a matter of course in most settings, as programmes need to maintain their environments and affairs. Cleaning up is not confined to food; after a messy craft activity, putting tables and chairs out and away again, and sweeping up, needs to be done. Some participants meet to attend to day-to-day business, such as planning for the month, rules and regulations, new policies, organising an outing and dealing with other issues that arise.

Recreational activities

There is always time for these. Playing games, putting on shows and going on trips are essential activities, although they are never the main focus of programmes. In one mental health programme, a game called 'Wheel of Fortune' has evolved and become an important tradition among those who have played it regularly for many years. The sheltered workshop has its own choir that meets for practice and performs regularly. The art workshop puts on exhibitions of work or performances such as an annual Wearable Arts show for mental health services.

Outings are a regular part of most of the programmes. Sometimes, they are to a particular event in the city or to the local swimming pool or golf driving range. Trips to the beach, the shopping mall or the gardens for a picnic and to feed the ducks are popular with mothers and children. Several programmes have an annual camp.

Special occasions

These are celebrated in many ways. Birthdays are usually acknowledged with a card, a song, a cake or a fuss of some kind. The midday meal may become something special or, at other times, people might go out for a meal to celebrate. Shows and performances may be part of a bigger celebration in which participants come together to reflect on what they have in common, for example, the tenth anniversary of the centre.

Time off for rest and relaxation

Little activities, such as having a quick smoke on the veranda, catching up on the gossip in the ladies' (or men's) room and making a quick phone call, can all oil the wheels of the programmes.

The practitioner

All the work being done is, in one way or another, related to the focus of the programme, and this is recognised by everyone. Some things are done out of necessity, because they need to be done, such as washing up or putting paper down on the table to protect it from paint spills. Other activities, for example bringing flowers for the lunch table, do not seem to fall into that category.

There are other activities that are not work at all, such as giving someone a hand with a task or noticing when someone does not turn up, which clearly provide a shared understanding among those who participate in a programme. We observed that everyone involved in a programme does these activities, including practitioners. What we noticed was that *everyone* belongs to the communities which exist in these settings and they all have complementary, and sometimes overlapping, parts to play in them.

Visible and invisible roles of the practitioner

Relationships are particularly clear within each setting and one thing that gives a clue to these is what people are called. The practitioner is rarely referred to by her professional title but is known as a manager, a supervisor, an artist or just by her own name. As with the work, the part each person plays is related to the focus of the setting. The relationships between people seem to reflect this, both formal production and general, daily life relationships. This appears to be why a *practitioner* so often seems to be invisible in these circumstances, through being a member of the community, with personal investment in it, just like anyone else.

However, the practitioner does have another role, which is implicitly rather than explicitly recognised. This involves much more than just her formal role in the community, although it depends on that role for its effectiveness. It guides what the practitioner does in the provision of the service and is dependent on her expertise. This invisible role, rather than the formal, visible role of manager or supervisor, is the practitioner's professional role.

Practitioner expertise

What often appears to be intuitive and pragmatic about the practitioner's actions in this invisible expert role is actually based on specific knowledge, skills and beliefs about how the world works, as well as on sound and necessary common sense. Briefly, this expertise seems to include:

Knowledge

- The meaning of community, how it comes about and the ongoing dynamics that sustain it;
- How things should be organised and the kind of facilitation and support necessary;
- Practical wisdom related to the mechanics of getting things done;
- Contextual knowledge and understanding of each individual's circumstances;
- Sound practical knowledge of how to do or make things – e.g. a card or a cake;
- Repertoire of activities, which can be categorised as food, craft and play;
- Many and varied resources and responses to draw on;
- The moral dilemmas of everyday life;
- Thorough local knowledge;
- Insight into the workings of the setting;
- How one thing leads to another – being able to let things happen while at the same time making sure the community continues to work;
- How some things arise naturally so that there are necessary things to do;
- How to deal with funding bodies, respond to structural change, report as required by law and protect the service from external pressures.

Skills

- Ability to ensure that people are *genuinely* and *naturally* occupied over extended periods of time;
- Ability to constantly make slight invisible adjustments to an activity to adapt to the needs of those taking part and ensure that it continues to work for its intended purpose;
- Ability to contribute to the management and administration of the service.

Attitudes

- Confidence in both the need for the service and its difference from other services;
- Commitment towards and genuine care for people;

- Belief in the right ways to go about things;
- Confidence in invisible/expert and visible/participant roles, and recognising when to take each one;
- Realistic view of how people get on, or not, in a community.

These knowledge, skills and attitudes have remained central to our understanding of the practitioner's role in these settings. These are the facts – the data – of practice. We will now consider the importance of language.

Language

In order not to be too removed from the world of practice, we want to use the language of the everyday. Starting with an intuitive idea that the words *occupant*, *occupation* and *occupy* describe well what is happening in our placement settings, we looked at them more closely. We became very observant about where these words appear, in conversation and in print, and how they are used. We checked out these usages and meanings with our students in class discussions. We also found that the *Oxford English Dictionary* (OED) (1989) (among many others, of course!) has already sorted and organised the various meanings of these terms, including some that we had not thought of. When we came to think about them, we agreed with all the dictionary entries because they capture the language we use when referring to our everyday experience.

The meaning of occupation

An occupant, or occupier, is the proper inhabitant of a place for which he has responsibility. Occupation consists in the results of living in an area, such as transformation of landscape, as well as processes such as economic activities. These activities might be what any inhabitant of a place (planet, country, suburb, house, apartment) would be involved in.

The idea that a person makes his own world is indicated by the way in which the word *occupation* is used to describe what happens when a country is occupied. All those activities that make the place a human habitation (as above) are controlled by the occupying power. Thus, active involvement in making this place theirs has been reduced for the inhabitants during this time, making them strangers in their own land.

People do not have to be occupied only by everyday business or trade, although we may be busy with these. We can also occupy ourselves with exploration, philosophical study or, as the *OED* points out, 'Whatever subject occupies discourse' too. We use the concept of being occupied in relation to ourselves when we are engaged in bringing about changes to the natural world. We can be occupied in imagining situations which are not present to the senses, or in distinguishing one part of nature from another and predicting how these parts might behave when they come into contact. We can be occupied with worrying about things or puzzling things out. We use the word *occupy* for those times when we are differentiating, connecting and constructing.

All this activity implies attention, and use of the word *occupied* frequently suggests engagement and close attention, particularly of the mind. Indeed, it often appears that minds and people are interchangeable when we talk of being occupied; that it is an individual (i.e. indivisible person) who does the occupying or is occupied. The implication is that this individual human being must attend so closely and engage so busily because his daily life is a great deal taken up with what he must do. This suggests that we need to occupy ourselves, all of ourselves, to attend to daily life in this way.

Distinguishing oneself as an individual, understanding oneself as a person, as human beings do, calls for very close attention if one is to seize and hold one's place in a world that, apparently, one must also construct. Our places, our positions, are held (we have tenure of them) by means of our craft and our work; familiar words that are both used in an occupational context. We use the noun *occupation* to describe our everyday business, employment or trade, all activities related to the material necessities of human life, as well as using the verb *occupy* to refer to our engagement in the process of bringing about these necessities.

All these meanings and usages of the words *occupant*, *occupation* and *occupy* come together to form a conceptual whole. *Occupation* refers quite literally to how people occupy and make the worlds that in turn, because we live in them, make and occupy us.

When we are occupied we are, in one way or another, doing *all* the things described above. Every time we use the words *occupation, occupant* and *occupy*, these meanings are inherent in what we say. This is why it is so important to be well occupied and to be, at some times, more (or less) occupied than at others.

We have found it useful to examine our everyday use of words, especially *occupy*. It is a good word, for it reminds us of our human condition: the disposition to change as well as use things, the need to make ourselves a home in the very particular human ways that we do and, in the process, to mind (in every way) what we are doing.

This examination of the first word in our professional title went a long way towards explaining what practitioners and participants are doing in the programmes where our students undertake their fieldwork placements. They are successfully making worlds to live in, in situations where this cannot be done without specific, and often ongoing, extra-ordinary support. A look back at how people are engaged in the placement settings described above shows why the words *occupant*, *occupation* and *occupy* are particularly applicable to what is being done there. These observations about the actual words we use indicate precisely what the focus of occupational practice should be: occupation as a domain of concern.

But apart from language as it is used for the practicalities of everyday life, there is also the language of literature which, by its very nature, is even more of an abstraction. Deliberate, intentional literary constructions give us a reflective, evaluative view of what humankind gets up to: ways to see ourselves and each other and to share our communal experience.

Literature

Wherever possible, we have left our illustrations as extracts from primary sources, firstly because we believe, with Burckhardt, in the eternal advantages referred to below and secondly because the way in which these sources substantiate and complement each other while speaking from different perspectives is seen more strongly this way. In every case, the sources from which these extracts come are worth reading in their entirety for the insights they bring to occupational practice.

> Now a source, as compared with a treatise, has its eternal advantages. First and foremost, it presents the fact pure, so that *we* must see what conclusions are to be drawn from it, while the treatise anticipates that labor and presents the fact digested, that is, placed in an alien, and often erroneous setting . . . beyond the labor we expend on sources the prize beckons in those great moments and fateful hours when, from things we have imagined long familiar, a sudden intuition dawns.
>
> (Burckhardt, 1945, pp. 52–3)

We have been fortunate that intuition has dawned many times as we have looked and re-looked at anthropological, imaginative, professional and other literature. But knowing which sources to go to is particularly important. The literature had to refer to the mundane activities of daily living *themselves* because it was these that needed explaining. Selecting sources from science as well as art seemed to be a good approach, since human beings have sought to know and understand the world by coming to it from both these fundamental perspectives.

In *The Educated Imagination*, Northrop Frye, a teacher, scholar and literary critic, distinguishes the arts from the sciences in the following way:

Science begins with the world we have to live in, accepting its data and trying to explain its laws. From there, it moves toward the imagination: it becomes a mental construct, a model of a possible way of interpreting experience. . . . Art, on the other hand, begins with the world we construct, not with the world we see. It starts with the imagination, and then works toward ordinary experience: that is, it tries to make itself as convincing and as recognizable as it can.

(Frye, 1964, p. 23)

The following few extracts from humanities literature have been chosen to illustrate, in a very elementary way, how science and art come together. They show us the way we make our worlds and sustain a human community identity through the everyday production of our means of subsistence, that is, through being occupied.

Anthropology

Anthropology is an obvious source to go to for this producing of the means to our subsistence because it provides theories about communities and how they are developed, structured and sustained. In *At Our Wit's Beginning*, Peter Wilson introduces some of the themes of anthropology, intending, he says, to convey some idea of what anthropology has discovered about 'the disguises and transformations, the masks and persona the human species has been trying on since its debut' (p. 1). He divides his monograph into three parts: *conceptions*, *connections* and *constructions*. Wilson says:

The human species survives because it adapts variously to the world via its societies and cultures. Selection operates upon these variations (in a sense it *is* these variations) and thereby the species evolves. So, to understand what human beings are, and to understand human evolution, we must investigate the nature, the structure, the organization and the function of human societies and human cultures, not simply as things in themselves, but as the products of the human species. We must connect them with the qualities and properties of the species for it is by this connection that individual specimens become *human* beings.

. . . as we begin, so does our world, for our world arises from our own conceptions, our ideas, theories, hypotheses and beliefs as our minds forever reach out ahead of and beyond our senses.

Conceived by and within nature the human species is a part of nature: *conceiving* of nature sets the species apart from nature. To verify our conceptions we set about exploring nature, making use of it to shore up our independence. Our ideas, explorations and use of nature *connects* us to the world, which also means to each other. As individuals we enjoy a measure of independence and individuality, but to prevent our being cast off we must rely upon our connections, our relationships, to sustain us. Having good connections, making connections, finding the right connections, are the ways in which human beings get on in the world.

Being connected to the world, conceiving of a world that is not apparent to our senses means that we join our ideas to the materials of the world and put a *construction* upon them and thereby build our own environments. In these we live within the environment of the world at large.

(Wilson, 1976, pp. 3–4)

These three dimensions of human nature – conception, connection and construction – speak strongly to our concept of occupation. Wilson's view of the way that human beings, having conceived of nature, must devise ways to connect with it as they construct it, is also manifested in the activities and relationships we observed in the placement settings. This again suggests, as a domain of concern those situations in which it is not possible for people to join their ideas to the materials of the world, put a construction on them and build their environments – where lack of good connections and relationships means isolation and idleness.

But how does all this conceiving, connecting and constructing get done in the ordinary way? How can we conceptualise what that consists in? Work, labour, craft and art are ideas that come to mind because they are words indicated by looking at our uses of *occupy* and *occupation*, and because they reflect what is going on in the placement settings too. For example, these words apply to the concentrated and committed effort which goes into economic activities: to the chores and repetitive tasks essential to keep places going; to the planning, strategising, figuring out and producing of desired results and also to all the little things they do, such as making the cake which was the centrepiece of a community celebration or the community art studio's Wearable Arts Show.

All these can, of course, be investigated by way of a number of disciplines as well as anthropology, and we have included only a few significant perspectives here; those that particularly illustrate what developed into a cultural view of occupation.

Work, labour, art and craft

Raymond Williams (1983) traced the meaning and usage of *work* and *labour* in his book about the words he considered key to the study of twentieth-century culture and society. Such dictionaries of culture were helpful in ensuring we were alert to distinctions being made when these words were used, especially when works have been translated, or written in a different period of time.

Philosopher and educationalist, T.F. Green, suggests three ways to consider the experience of work for human beings. They relate very closely to those situations for which we use the words occupy and occupation. Briefly summarised (drawn from Green, 1968, chapters 2 and 3), these are:

- **Labour**: Mere activity characterised by necessity and futility. The goods produced by labour are consumed and have no enduring quality. A man is not free whose life is totally absorbed in labour. His energies are spent in response to necessity, under the aegis of forces outside himself, forces he cannot control. He is not master of himself as he is himself mastered.

- **Job**: The occupation which one does for pay. It may be seen as obligatory and done of necessity (labour) and/or engendering activity which is purposeful and meaningful to the individual (work).

- **Work**: Activity producing an enduring object. Work requires self-investment, skill, craft and personal judgement. Work is purposeful *and* meaningful. Work is distinct from labour and often must be discovered independently from one's job.

However, Green also makes some interesting observations about the seemingly futile and repetitive chores of life, which illustrate his view of the significance of community and identity in the ordinary things we do. This is particularly relevant to our placement programmes, for example, in putting flowers on the lunch table and washing up.

> [labours of love]. The fact, however, [is] the difference love makes, the difference in seeing a task in one's 'sensed community', as part of one's own 'creation', 'imagination', and 'autobiography' . . . Setting the table three times a day with the bunny plate for Jean and the special blueberry muffin for John becomes something more than a transient and fleeting achievement. It takes on the character of a durable thing: not simply setting the table, which is of course undone, but setting it for this particular Jean or John, at this particular age and inclination. (p. 26)
>
> Indeed, at times when people's energies are required in order to satisfy some obviously fundamental human needs, they do not even ask whether their work is justified. . . . The proper response to anyone who might ask whether such work is justified would be simply to show him what needs doing. Beyond that recognition, no recognition, no justification is possible or needed, and indeed the question, 'Of what good is it?' would not even arise. (Green, 1968, p. 41)

Erich Fromm, in this extract from *Escape from Freedom*, sees love and work together as essential if the individual and his world are to be united in forming a human/natural whole.

> Spontaneous activity is the one way in which man can overcome the terror of aloneness without sacrificing the integrity of his self . . . Love is the foremost component of such spontaneity; not love as the dissolution of the self in another person, but love as spontaneous affirmation of others, as the union of the individual with others on the basis of the preservation of the individual self. . . . Work is the other component; not work as a compulsive activity in order to escape aloneness, not work as a relationship to nature which is partly one of dominating her, partly one of worship of and enslavement by the very products of man's hands, but work as creation in which man becomes one with nature in the act of creation. What holds true of love and work holds true of all spontaneous action . . . It affirms the individuality of the self and at the same time it unites the self with man and nature.
>
> (Fromm, 1972, p. 260)

This spontaneous work in which people become one with nature and other human beings in an act of creation reminds us of views such as Ernst Fischer's idea of the necessity of art:

> Evidently man wants to be more than just himself. He wants to be a *whole* man. He is not satisfied with being a separate individual . . . what a man apprehends as his potential includes everything that humanity as a whole is capable of. Art is the indispensable means for this merging of the individual in the whole. It reflects his infinite capacity for association, for sharing experiences and ideas.
>
> (Fischer, 1978, pp. 8–9)

The artists (including staff) at our art studio placement in Dunedin demonstrate an understanding of this art, in particular its fundamentally associative character, but so also, in seemingly small but significant ways, do those in all the placement settings described above. Through daily labours of love, bonds are made that bring into being the communities that then sustain them.

So what of craft? This has always been an important concept for us, because its essence – seeing the possibilities in situations, or alternative strategies that we might pursue to achieve an end or solve a problem – is fundamental to humankind's occupation of our planet, as we have seen above. It is also strongly associated with our professional heritage.

We could not get on or feel at home in our world if we could not make decisions about what to do, express ourselves in creative ways and understand each other. This resourcefulness, this craft, requires the utmost attention to what people are doing, to what is going on. It must be discriminating and careful, yet bold and daring. It must anticipate, be mindful of the consequences, consider what *could* happen. And although a crafty man is considered to be a bit devious, deceitful even in solving his problems, the idea of a craftsman embodies all that is good, that is creative yet respectful of tradition, in human action or work. The literature of craft, whether craftspeople's own accounts or philosophies of craft, tells in great detail the history of humankind, that crafty and caring conceiver, connector and constructor. Being occupied has everything to do with craft.

In *The Principles of Art*, R.G. Collingwood defines craft as 'the power to produce a preconceived result by means of consciously controlled and directed action' (1958, p. 15). In one of the most quoted passages from *Capital*, Marx describes the work required to realise this power:

> We presuppose labour in a form that stamps it as exclusively human. A spider conducts operations that resemble those of the weaver; and a bee puts to shame many an architect in the construction of her cells. But what distinguishes the worst architect from the best of bees is this, that the architect raises his structure in imagination before he erects it in reality. At the end of every labour-process, we get a result that already existed in the imagination of the labourer at its commencement. He not only effects a change of form in the material on which he works, but he also realises a purpose of his own that gives the law to his modus operandi, and to which he must subordinate his will. And this subordination is no mere momentary act. Besides the exertion of the bodily organs, the process demands that, during the whole operation, the workman's will be steadily in consonance with his purpose. This means close attention.
>
> (Marx, 1912, p. 156)

Imagination, close attention, work, labour, art, craft, conceptions, connections and constructions: these concepts illustrate why anthropology is such a key discipline in our understanding of occupation. Anthropology is about the things people do that create the connections and constructions which form the purposes and make the meaning. This is well illustrated by the following extract from Margaret Visser's (1989) anthropological analysis of humankind's ways with food. As shown above, food is a key component of the work done in all our placement communities.

Food is 'everyday' – it has to be, or we would not survive for long. But food is never just something to eat. It is something to find or hunt or cultivate first of all; for most of human history we have spent a much longer portion of our lives worrying about food, and plotting, working, and fighting to obtain it, than we have in any other pursuit. As soon as we can count on a food supply (and so take food for granted), and not a moment sooner, we start to civilise ourselves. Civilisation entails shaping, regulating, constraining, and dramatising ourselves; we echo the preferences and the principles of our culture in the way we treat our food. An elaborate frozen dessert moulded into the shape of a ruined classical temple can be read as one vivid expression of a society's view of itself and its ideals; so can a round ground hamburger patty between two circular buns. Food – what is chosen from the possibilities available, how it is presented, how it is eaten, with whom and when, and how much time is allotted to cooking and eating it – is one of the means by which a society creates itself and acts out its aims and fantasies. Changing (or unchanging) food choices and presentations are part of every society's tradition and character. Food shapes us and expresses us even more definitively than our houses or utensils do.

(Visser, 1989, p. 12)

Thus, the interpretations and propositions of anthropology, and philosophies of art, craft, work and labour, give us a substantial picture of the what, the how and the wherefore of occupation and insights into what our placement programmes are all about. But these insights are into the conditions of human existence; the world we see, as Northrop Frye says. To get the other side of the picture, an inside view of what it is to be a human being, making and making our way in the world, we had to go to the imaginative constructions of humankind.

Imaginative literature

No written form except imaginative literature comes even close to giving us an understanding of human individuals within their own creation, their 'sensed community' as Green (1968) puts it. Of course, personal accounts of experience can be extremely valuable, but imaginative literature speaks not of the experience of particular people but of what it is to be part of humanity itself. Imaginative literature sources contribute not only to the body of knowledge a practitioner needs to *deliver* his or her service but also to the understanding he or she needs both to *recognise* and to *offer* it.

The simple point is that literature belongs to the world man constructs, not to the world he sees; to his home, not his environment. Literature's world is a concrete human world of immediate experience. The poet uses images and objects and sensations much more than he does abstract ideas; the novelist is concerned with telling stories, not with working out arguments. The world of literature is human in shape, a world where the sun rises in the east and sets in the west over the edge of a flat earth in three dimensions, where the primary realities are not atoms or electrons but bodies, and the primary forces not energy or gravitation but love and death and passion and joy.

(Frye, 1964, pp. 27–8)

The practitioners we have observed over the years appear to have a very good grasp of the 'world man constructs . . . his home', and they are intimately involved in making sure that those they work with participate fully in it. But this concrete, human world of immediate experience is one that both practitioner and partici-pant share so *both* must, in some part, respond to the primary forces of love and death and passion and joy.

Northrop Frye suggests that 'the story of the loss and regaining of identity is the framework of all literature' (1964, p. 55). Sustaining identity is something that people in our placement settings are doing (with the help they need) through the ordinary everyday tasks done as part of their 'sensed community'. Because of this, imaginative literature has helped to keep us close to the real, concrete human world of practice. A few extracts follow, drawn from imaginative literature, which speak to this world as we came to know and understand it.

The Grapes of Wrath is John Steinbeck's story of dispossessed Oklahoma farmers and their life-and-death struggle to find a new home in California. For much of the time they are in transit. It is a story of human endurance, of hope and despair, work and love.

The cars of the migrant people crawled out of the side roads on to the great cross-country highway . . . and as the dark caught them, they clustered like bugs near to shelter and to water. And because they were lonely and perplexed, because they had all come from a place of sadness and worry and defeat, and because they were all going to a mysterious place, they huddled together; they talked together; they shared their lives, their food and the things they hoped for . . . At first the families were timid in the building and tumbling worlds, but gradually the technique of building worlds became their technique. Then leaders emerged, then laws were made, then codes came into being. And as the worlds moved westwards they were more complete and better furnished, for their builders were more experienced in building them . . . And the worlds were built in the evening. The people, moving from the highways, made them with their tents and their hearts and their brains . . . Thus they changed their social life – changed as in the whole universe only men can change.

(Steinbeck, 1993, chapter 10)

The way that human community is a matter of making worlds through people's own effort is seen in the following extract from *Potiki*, by Patricia Grace. Here, the relationship between the made and the maker, past and present, is conceived as parts of an organic whole which is constantly building and rebuilding itself.

We were all caught up in the excitement of planning, building and decorating the new house, of working out designs and patterns, and watching these grow. Some of the patterns and designs followed the old ones, these being already part of ourselves. They were etched on the memory and were patterns of the stars and the sea, of the fish and birds and plants, and also of learning and relationships, conflict, sorrow and joy. But there were new patterns too, of flooding and fire, roads and machines, oneness and strength, and work and growth.

We were caught up, both in the excitement, and in the exhaustion of working from daybreak until dark, and then after dark. Because there were still the gardens to work during daylight hours and still the fishing to be done, although I could not, by then, go fishing or work on the land, and was not allowed to exhaust myself the ways that others did.

'Build something, and it builds you,' was what Hoani said, and I thought of a long time ago when the old lady had said to me, 'You know what I do, I make myself.' And she had given me the little kit which I have still. 'It's myself, to give,' she'd said. 'And your big fish, it's yourself, to give.'

(Grace, 1986, pp. 143–4)

A Work of Art, by Margaret Mahy, is a story of what seems a very ordinary affair – a mother making a birthday cake for her son. It is indeed very ordinary, the sort of activity which orders our days, and Mrs Baskin herself goes about her task in a required order also. But there is more to birthday cake making than technical order. Order is given to the days of Mrs Baskin's whole family through the making of this cake. Through it, many things are brought together in a recognisable, meaningful way. Through Mrs Baskin's cake, many come together as one – and are very well aware that they have done so.

Mrs Baskin set about things in a very orderly fashion. First she greased one side of the greaseproof paper with a knob of butter, and then she fitted it, butter side up, in the big, hinged cake tin. She turned on the oven so that it would be heating while she worked. Then she put the dried fruit into the plastic bowl – currants, candied peel, sultanas, seedless raisins, a little bit of chopped ginger and almonds, as well as glacé cherries and crystallized angelica to give a bit of colour to the cake when it was sliced. Once she'd mixed the dried fruit, she floured it a little so the fruit wouldn't stick to itself. Then she sifted half a pound of plain flour and half a teaspoon of baking powder into yet another bowl, an old pottery one that had belonged to her mother.

Her three youngest children, Hamlet, Serena and Toby, watched her, for they were as interested in Brian's cake as if it were theirs too. They were certain Brian would let them have some of it. Even Wellington, the dog, watched, wagging his tail whenever anyone spoke to him. Hubert, the cat, pretended to be asleep, but if you looked closely you could see two thin, green slits in his black face. He liked to know just what was going on in his house.

(Mahy, 1988, pp. 36–7)

... Mrs Baskin ... made herself a cup of tea, turned the television off, and sat in the moony dark for a little while, getting herself into a magical, cake icing mood. She had a short, refreshing sleep, then got up, washed her face and put on some make-up (so as to get in a birthday party mood). She thought about Brian who had been her first baby. She thought about him growing year by year, losing teeth, scraping his knees, learning how to ride a bike, going to college, and so on. The cake needed to be iced in such a way that anyone who saw it would somehow be aware of these things. She would not write *Happy Birthday* on it but she would ice it so that anyone who saw it would *feel* Happy Birthday-ish.

(Mahy, 1988, p. 39)

In Lionel Trilling's chilling novel of estrangement in everyday life, *The Middle of the Journey* (the allusion in the title to Dante's *Inferno* is apt), there is one of the most poignant illustrations of the fragility of human identity. Here, old Mr Folger's defence of his family's existence in battle is repaid by their defence of his existence as they see to it that he can still perform his duty.

Old Mr. Folger was so on the edge of life that he was scarcely a person any longer, yet he was kept a person by his inclusion here, by the little duties he performed, such as this one of fetching the eggs. It was impossible to believe that he had stood at Gettysburg, but he had indeed.

(Trilling, 1957, p. 72)

J.R.R. Tolkien has Bilbo, Gandalf, and Thorin Oakenshield's company of dwarves rest and recuperate at the Last Homely House in the West, that of Elrond the Elf-friend, on their way to the Lonely Mountain.

His house was perfect, whether you liked food, or sleep, or work, or story-telling, or singing, or just sitting and thinking best, or a pleasant mixture of them all.

(Tolkien, 1996, chapter 3)

Elrond's house is a highly cultured haven. It is not the world that men and hobbits will inherit after the last War of the Ring but a vision of cultivated perfection, the recipe for which they will need to keep alive and be able to recreate, at least in some part, for themselves when their own recreation is needed (as of course it will be). This is a little like the recreation that reconstruction aides were expected to be part of, away back at the dawn of our profession, or in the early days of moral treatment, or perhaps even now in community programmes in Dunedin.

These tiny illustrations have not even touched on the understandings we gained from myths, legends, fantasy and science fiction: stories of the great and glorious, the honest and true, the cunning and devious and the way we all began. These imaginative constructions tell of what humankind gets up to, of how we make our worlds go round all over the globe and have done so since the beginning of time. Such stories, of course, are part of the heritage of our practice communities, known and told and loved by most in one form or another. And apart from the general human truths which they impart, a practitioner needs to be familiar with these traditional, canonical stories because they are the means by which we come together in coming to terms with our common human experience. If we know our own myths and legends, we know what it is to have them as part of who we are.

Which bring us to what has been written about our professional practice.

Professional literature

We had a clear idea about where our focus came from – its provenance – from reading our professional literature. We give three examples here to illustrate this idea, one from our New Zealand professional history (1940s), one from the *American Journal of Occupational Therapy* (1971), and one from the World Federation of Occupational Therapists (2002).

In her account of the beginnings of occupational therapy in New Zealand, Hazel Skilton writes about the work going on at the Auckland Mental Hospital in the 1940s and in New Caledonia during the Second World War. This work, craft and community focus has continued in many settings in New Zealand ever since, surviving the sometimes quite traumatic effects of government policy changes in service delivery. Just as in our Dunedin practice settings, there is a focus on the work needing to be done and on the way in which being involved in these purposeful, one-thing-leads-to-another, collaborative and co-operative enterprises raises confidence, improves morale and creates meaning, thereby encouraging reconstruction, recreation and recuperation. Physical and mental capabilities (together with any psychological effects of injury) were very practically, and often most ingeniously, taken account of, but always carefully and with great sensitivity.

The carpenter patient made suggestions for the layout of the workshop, and set the men to work putting up benches and arranging tools. One of Charlie's (the male nurse) friends gave him a woodturning lathe and this was set up. Now that the patients had become used to 'going to work' each day, and had proved just what they could do with a little help and encouragement, it was thought that even woodturning was possible. This lathe proved a boon. It greatly widened the scope of articles that could be made, such as sturdy stool frames. These were glued and cramped together by another group of patients, and the tops were woven in patterns in seagrass. Dangerous tools, such as electric drills, planers and saws were kept inside an area protected by a wire netting fence. (p. 38)

  . . . one man . . . used to make regular visits to the Meola Tip, returning with a haul of bits of machinery, pieces of metal, the wildest collection of old junk imaginable. From these he patiently fashioned exquisitely made tools. Some of these machines were capable of making the finest precision tools, which were invaluable in engineering projects involving other patients.

(Skilton, 1981, p. 39)

And in New Caledonia, 1944:

The accommodation provided for the occupational therapy department was excellent . . . but all the Quartermaster could supply in the way of equipment was trestle tables and stools. He did arrange, though, that two crashed aeroplanes would be delivered to her!! . . . those planes were a challenge though. Some of the patients had a few tools of their own, among them hacksaw blades, but alas, no frames to hold them. However, frames were eventually made from piping salvaged from the planes. These were more like museum pieces than works of art, but they served the purpose. Now it was possible to cut stainless steel and duralium from the planes and use this for the manufacture of various types of souvenir. Two patients even made an ingenious treadle wood-turning lathe from the planes' roller bearings, two ends of wire drums riveted together to form a wheel, and a packing case converted into a table. The result was most satisfactory. The local woods proved very suitable for wood-turning, as well as for carving and polishing. Perspex from the panes was also used to make salad servers, butter knives and other small articles.

(Skilton, 1981, pp. 50–1)

Almost 30 years later, in 1971, Dr Bockhoven wrote in the *American Journal of Occupational Therapy* of his belief that the history of moral treatment (at least in the United States) is also the history of occupational therapy. This assertion, he says, is based on the idea that occupational therapy is based first and foremost on respect for human individuality and on a fundamental perception of a person's need to engage in creative activity in relation to his fellow man. It shows very clearly a belief that people make themselves as they make the world, and their place within it, and that enabling people to do this is what occupational therapy consists in. He explains that the philosophy of moral treatment:

> ... based on the faith that the 'mentally deranged person can best recover his reason in the company of persons of sound mind and kindly nature who would help him by joining with him in the regimen of daily life.'
> The 'regimen of daily life,' it should be noted with special attention by today's occupational therapist, consisted of creative and recreational activity with others. The early-day moral treatment hospitals were equipped with a variety of craft shops and recreational areas indoors. The grounds outside the building were divided into garden areas and outdoor game areas. These areas were in turn surrounded by farmland under active cultivation and with diversi-fied agriculture.
> It appears almost conspicuously evident that moral treatment could be reasonably described in philosophy and practice as a comprehensive occupational therapy program ... Without meaningful synchronized produc-tive interchange with others there tends to be nothing but fanciful, hypo-thetical, abstract as-if-ism in our preventive, therapeutic and rehabilitative endeavours.

Bockhoven insists that such endevors are:

> ... cultural processes that depend on loving cultivation and careful atten-tion to supplying prerequisites such as accessible learning experiences and sufficient time for them to be absorbed, integrated, and applied.
> ... It is the occupational therapist's inborn respect for the realities of life, for the real tasks of living, and the time it takes the individual to develop his modes of coping with his tasks, that leads me to urge haste on the profession of occupational therapy to assert its leadership in fashioning the design of human services programs.
> Perhaps no other discipline is likely to have this perspective for occupa-tional therapy is almost the only remaining discipline that has more respect for people in their actual situations than for fanciful pet ideas about human behaviour.
> (Bockhoven, 1971, pp. 223–5)

Bockhoven mentions the 'regimen of daily life . . . creative and recreational activity with others', for example, craft shops, garden areas, outdoor games and active cultivation of farmland: 'meaningful synchronized productive interchange with others'. He emphasises that the changes people must make are 'cultural processes that depend on loving cultivation and careful attention' and that, as such, they require 'accessible learning experiences' and 'time to be absorbed, integrated and applied'. This choice of words underlines an understanding of occupation as a cultural concept rather than a psychological or physical one, and that being well occupied is a matter of experience, and experience invariably requires time.

Thirty years after Bockhoven offered this advice, the World Federation of Occupational Therapists' *Revised Minimum Standards for the Education of Occupational Therapists* (2002) advises that:

> Programmes for the education of occupational therapists are guided by a unique philosophical understanding of occupation, derived from a unique mix of international and local perspectives and understandings. . . . The programme's philosophical understanding of occupation may include:
>
> 1. the nature and meaning of occupation
> 2. the occupational nature of humans
> 3. the kinds of problems and satisfactions people experience in relation to participating in occupation
> 4. cultural understandings about how problems with participation in occupation might be addressed and how the experience or outcomes of participation might be enhanced.
>
> (World Federation of Occupational Therapists, 2002)

As well as advising that we should be certain of our philosophical assumptions, the document encourages us to look to our professional heritage and our local context. This we have done consistently throughout the years since the beginning of the undergraduate programme. Our heritage is alluded to above, as is our local context, which includes our practice placements. So too is our investigation of the nature and meaning of occupation through the usage of the word itself and in the literature of the humanities.

Discussion

These overall understandings have been invaluable in helping us to recognise needs (of both client and practitioner) in a much more discriminating way and also to begin constructing basic frames of reference which can help to guide the practice of students (and, we have found, practitioners too) in specific settings.

Through making these connections ourselves, we have come to understand some things that are often troubling when trying to explain what an occupational therapist does and why. Our title speaks to a basic human need and we have never found any word other than *occupation* that can do this as well. And it is used every day, which is why people know that occupational therapists keep people occupied by giving them something to do: something that is *for* something, that has a point, a purpose, a meaning. Being occupied is putting our minds to something and doing it. It is having something to do that contributes to the practical human world, to the exploration and discovery of things about the world we see, and/or to the imaginary world we construct – through work, labour, craft and art.

We can now begin to explain, for example, that therapy is not just about what the client wants to do. Over the years, there has too often been a focus on getting people to 'make up their own minds' and to 'decide for themselves'. This seems to be an extraordinary approach when, in so many contexts, knowing what to do is precisely the problem.

Build something and it builds you: 'the activity told me what to do'. Gardening and produce, cakes and jam, Christmas trees and reusing buttons, buying, selling and exchanging keep us grounded, in touch, but they cultivate us too. When you lack confidence, doubt your worth, feel estranged and disenfranchised, the last thing you can do is be crafty, creative, concerned and responsible on your own. What you need is for there to be something (and not necessarily always someone) that will tell you what to do for as long as you need. This is why those soldiers were making souvenirs out of crashed aeroplanes and why everyone takes turns with washing up, making cakes and birthday cards, mowing the lawns and fetching the eggs. Occupational practitioners bring people and the world back together and, because people must in reality do this themselves, the contexts must be real and immediate. This is what the souvenirs in New Caledonia were for. They had to be made or else demand from the market would not be met – and salad servers, butter knives, birthday cards or midday meals will not make themselves. They require the power to produce a preconceived result by means of consciously controlled and directed action. To have that power is craft; to exercise it is work. To exercise it is to be, in this case, well occupied, for at least as long as the work lasts.

Our practitioners understand that for different sorts of reasons people often have nowhere to go and nothing to do. If they were able to find or create a place of their own where they *do* have something to do, programmes like these would not be necessary. Practitioners also believe that daily life and work are built and sustained through people's own actions, and that much of their confidence and identity derives from this. They know that what is needed is real work, everyday chores, rest and recreation through which meaning and purpose can be found.

They also know how difficult this is for participants, who need help and often ongoing support. And that is what they were clearly doing: caringly and consistently supporting people in their *own* creation and maintenance of daily life and work.

There are many situations in everyday human life, at work, at home, as citizens, where our occupations are managed by someone other than ourselves. But mostly we keep ourselves occupied, because of the work we engage in and, in doing so, find help where and when we need it. But when one is charged, as these practitioners are, with the responsibility for keeping another person occupied, in other words, helping him make the world wherein he makes himself, the guidance of Scheffler's (1985) ethical ideal is of particular concern. There are two very clear ethical points to be made.

First, if one is to be responsible for keeping a person occupied (since it is not, in the circumstances, possible for them to do so by themselves), it must be the person's occupation, and not the occupation of the practitioner, which is the focus. Where this is happening, the service providers (the practitioners) are of necessity invisible. They cannot be occupied *instead of* the person any more than the nurse should *drink the milk* for the undernourished child or the teacher *learn to read* for the student. But the processes of nursing or teaching readily allow for a visible helpmeet. Human beings acknowledge their dependence on precept and know that they must depend on others for food when they are very young. And if you postulate an end then the means will always have disappeared when the end is reached: that is why it is called the end. This is the nature of a means/end relationship. So, if a practitioner is the means to a client's end, she will always do herself out of a job if she is successful. These practitioners are in the business of *keeping* people well occupied and if that is happening the way it should it is the practitioner's destiny to remain invisible throughout.

However, as we discovered from our practice observations, the occupational practitioner must be an invisible *practitioner* but not an invisible *participant* in this cultural context that is the domain of concern. She must be a true participant and not remain aloof or remote within that cultural context. If people are successfully being kept occupied, the scene should resemble any other where people are well occupied, despite there being particular difficulties pertaining to it.

Second, it matters a great deal what the person is being occupied by. Things must be made or done well, which is why work must not be foolish, busy work. There must be a real point to it. It must be required to be finished and it must be done properly, that is, to the standard required for the purpose. The heart of moral treatment is not just *treating* someone with respect, it is showing that respect by providing the opportunity for people to be responsible, careful, respectful and mindful *themselves*, and being there to help when necessary. That means giving people worthwhile things to do – as Bockhoven points out, and as Hazel Skilton (1981) and our practitioners illustrate.

Conclusion

Our intention when we began to search, by various means, for an explanation of what goes on in our student community placement settings was to find something which would guide our delivery of undergraduate education. We started from observations of the practice we wanted to explain.

In the contexts in which this practice is going on, people are doing all manner of ordinary things, in the course of which they puzzle and plan, investigate and explore. They show and tell, look and listen. They philosophise, contemplate and ponder. They investigate, explore, debate and discuss, think, imagine and wonder. In short they conceptualise, connect and construct everything from their love lives and lunches to life, the universe and everything, even though that is often not at all easy to do.

What these observations highlighted for us was that:

1. work, labour, art and craft are important in all of the settings;
2. an idea of community is present in all of them;
3. people themselves are *making things happen*;
4. *making things happen* cannot be done without support;
5. the practitioner has an invisible expert role, as well as a visible participant one.

In our search for an explanation for what is going on, so that we could fulfil our obligation as the educators of such practitioners (and, more recently to provide a justification for the ongoing provision of such services), we made connections between what we were observing, the concept of occupation and literature sources, both disciplinary and imaginary. As time and our connections became stronger we become certain that:

6. the best way to express this practice is through the language of culture;
7. culture is the foundation of occupational practice, and not just something to take into account because the people with whom we work 'come' from one culture or another;
8. we should understand culture because the result of human occupation *is* culture;

9. the philosophical assumption behind this, our domain of concern, is that, like it or not, for good and for ill, *humankind makes itself*;

10. anthropology is a key discipline to capture the rational approach to human culture;

11. imaginative forms of expression capture the aesthetic and moral dimensions of human culture.

When exploring our professional provenance, we discovered that this orientation has been and continues to be reflected in our professional stories and literature.

It is more than a little strange, but also gratifying, to remind ourselves that the situation we had at the beginning, was that:

1. services were being provided to meet an ongoing need for activity and community integration;

2. the focus of all these services was occupation;

3. we were occupational therapists (or occupational practitioners).

Well, now we have found some ways which articulate, and also go some way towards explaining, that.

Without suggesting that all occupational therapists will find this view a useful one to explain their practice, it has been a most useful one for us. It offers the possibility of identifying a broad domain of concern and various problems of ordinary experience within it. It also suggests what knowledge and skills are needed for the job if it is always to be done well.

We are no longer obliged to use the word *occupation* in every sentence we utter. The words *occupy* and *occupation* often arise quite naturally, of course, but usually we are able freely to speak about mind and attention, work and craft, art and labour and community – and their interrelationship – and know that not only does everyone understand one another but also that we are all always on track. Mainly this is because we are all speaking the language of ordinary experience. We count ourselves lucky that since our domain of concern is the everyday, our specialised professional vocabulary must also necessarily come from that same language.

References

Bockhoven, J.S. (1971) Legacy of Moral Treatment: 1800s–1910. *American Journal of Occupational Therapy.* **25**(5): 223–5.

Burckhardt, J. (1945) *Reflections on History* (trans. M.D. Hottinger), Liberty Classics, Indianapolis (original lectures given between 1868 and 1885; expanded in 1941 by Werner Kägi).

Collingwood, R.G. (1958) *The Principles of Art*, Oxford University Press, Oxford (original work published 1938).

Fischer, E. (1978) *The Necessity of Art* (trans. Anna Bostock), Penguin Peregrine, London (original work published 1959).

Fromm, Erich (1972) *Escape from Freedom*, Holt, Rinehart & Winston, New York (original work published 1941).

Frye, N. (1964) *The Educated Imagination*, Indiana University Press, Bloomington, IN.

Grace, P. (1986) *Potiki*, Penguin Books, Auckland, New Zealand.

Green, T.F. (1968) *Work, Leisure and the American Schools*, Random House, New York.

Mahy, M. (1988) A work of art, in *The Door in the Air and Other Stories*, J.M. Dent & Sons, London.

Marx, K. (1912) *Capital* (trans. S. Moore and E. Aveling), William Glaisher, London (original work published 1886).

Mosey, A.C. (1985) *Configuration of a Profession*, Raven Press, New York.

Oxford English Dictionary (1989) Clarendon Press, Oxford.

Scheffler, I. (1985) *Of Human Potential*, Routledge & Kegan Paul, Boston, MA.

Skilton, H. (1981) *Work for your Life: The Story of the Beginning and Early Years of Occupational Therapy in New Zealand*, Hudlo Printers, Hamilton.

Steinbeck, J. (1993) *The Grapes of Wrath*, Minerva, London (original work published 1939).

Tolkien, J.R.R. (1996) *The Hobbit: Or There and Back Again*, HarperCollins, London (original work published 1937).

Trilling, L. (1957) *The Middle of the Journey*, Doubleday Anchor Books, New York.

Visser, M. (1989) *Much Depends on Dinner*, Penguin, London.

Williams, R. (1983) *Keywords: A Vocabulary of Culture and Society*, 2nd edn, Fontana Press, London.

Wilson, P.J. (1976) *At Our Wits Beginning*, Anthropology Department, Otago University, Dunedin, New Zealand.

World Federation of Occupational Therapists (2002) *Revised Minimum Standards for the Education of Occupational Therapists*, WFOT (wfot@multiline.com.au).

When service users' views vary from those of their carers

6

Elizabeth White

Introduction

One of the skills that marks out an expert occupational therapist is his or her ability to engage with each service user as an individual living within their own environment. Such a skill enables the therapist to act in a client-focused way, identifying the activities that are meaningful and relevant to each person and working in partnership to devise therapeutic interventions that are individually tailored to reach the desired goals.

The overarching aim of occupational therapy, according to Creek (2003) is to

> maintain, restore or create a match, beneficial to the individual, between the abilities of the person, the demands of his/her occupations in the areas of self-care, productivity and leisure, and the demands of the environment.
>
> (Creek, 2003, p. 8)

This view clearly places the service user at the centre of intervention planning, suggesting a negotiated approach between the desires of the individual, the limitations or opportunities afforded by their disability and external environments, and the skills and knowledge of the therapist.

The purpose of this chapter is to discuss the findings of a research study designed to explore the multifaceted, and at times conflicting, factors that confront and influence the therapist in her clinical decision-making in the setting of a wheelchair seating clinic. The complex nature of the disabilities of service users who require supportive seating, and their level of dependency and consequent reliance on a range of carers, provide a challenging scenario for the therapist. Equipment provision may aim to prioritise the identified or perceived needs of the service user, but achieving occupational engagement can be significantly influenced by the abilities, perspectives and motivation of carers. An additional dimension occurs when service users have impaired or absent verbal communication, as ascertaining their own views and preferences can then be extremely difficult. Yet there should be no assumption that a carer or other representative can accurately provide such information on their behalf.

The partnership between people with disabilities and their carers

Aiming for the acquisition of skills that enable a person with a disability to achieve independence in their chosen activities may be the ultimate goal for therapist and service user alike. The reality is that many people have congenital or acquired impairments that impact on their ability to lead lives in which they are not dependent on someone else for some part of their personal care or social, work or educational needs. Practical assistance may be given by paid helpers or by friends and family members, and the Department of Health (2006) estimates that there are some 5.7 million carers in Britain, most of them middle-aged or older.

Paying attention to carers' needs and demands is an integral part of occupational therapy practice (Turner *et al.*, 2002) and requires consideration of the physical, psychological, emotional and financial impact of caring for someone with disabilities. Arguably, the greater the level of impairment experienced by the disabled person, the more profound will be the impact on carers' lives. Occupational therapists routinely involve carers when planning their therapeutic interventions, and consider the level of support that can be offered in pursuit of the desired goals. Thus, the outcome for a service user with an enduring disability may be framed by the boundaries of his or her carer's abilities and attitudes.

What occupational therapists may be less focused on, however, are the perspectives of both service users and their carers towards the impact and implications of the caring role on long-term health and quality of life for both partners. The reality of an ageing population, with many carers themselves being elderly or having health difficulties, and the physically demanding nature of caring for someone with physical disabilities, presents a situation in which both the carer and the cared-for may have an acute awareness of potentially harmful long-term outcomes. Wear and tear on the carer or a diminution of quality of healthy, meaningful living on the part of the disabled person may both be likely scenarios. In a relationship where the disabled person and his or her carer have a strong emotional attachment, such as between marital partners or a parent and child, a considerable level of guilt may be attached to a caring relationship. The disabled partner can feel guilty about the burdensome nature of their needs and desires, while the carer may feel resentful of the demands made on their physical resources and the restrictions that may be placed on their own activities.

Do occupational therapists acknowledge this scenario and elicit the views of their service users and carers on what they both want to achieve when planning interventions? Or is the seemingly inevitable mismatch between a disabled person's need for meaningful lived experiences and their carer's physical and emotional capacity an insoluble conundrum that is beyond the therapist's brief? Some insight into the dilemma was revealed during an ethnographic study of severely physically disabled people.

The ethnographic study

This study took place within the multidisciplinary setting of a wheelchair clinic, an environment within which services users, professional and family carers, and a range of health, social care and education professionals interacted. The study group comprised 19 people across all ages with a congenital, acquired or learning disability, all of whom were users of wheelchairs with special seating systems. Observations made during the wheelchair clinic sessions were supplemented by key themes underpinning wheelchair seating provision that had been derived from a literature review and participant case notes. From this information, the researcher developed a semi-structured interview schedule that allowed a more detailed exploration of the role and importance of wheelchair seating with the sampled service users, their carers and the professional staff who worked closely with them.

It is estimated that some 10% of wheelchair users in the United Kingdom require special seating in order to provide the postural support that is necessary to maintain a sitting position while using a wheelchair (British Society of Rehabilitation Medicine, 1995), and this population includes some of the most severely physically disabled people with whom occupational therapists work. In the wheelchair clinic, the breadth of experience and expertise that was accessible during appointments enabled all contexts within which the wheelchair and seating system were used to be included in discussions and prescription processes. By placing the needs of the service user at the centre of decision making, physical, psychosocial and environmental factors could all be recognised and maximum benefit afforded from the equipment that was provided.

Given the severity of disability experienced by the service users, and the complexity of their needs, the wheelchairs and seating systems supplied as outcomes of the clinic assessment were correspondingly complex. Implications for carers were the handling and management of equipment that could be heavy and bulky, requiring a clear understanding of correct application, and a certain level of physical ability and technical dexterity. A particular impact was noted on transportation needs, with many of the service users having such postural and transferring difficulties that it was essential for them to be transported in their wheelchair and seating system. A further dimension was added with the number of accessories required to enable the user to undertake a range of activities, given that the wheelchair formed the main mode for sitting during the day.

At an early stage of the researcher's observations it was apparent that there was a lack of congruence in the approaches of the various participants within the clinic setting, and the desired outcomes were differently prioritised. While clinical need was acknowledged as being the foundation on which decision making should be based, the service users' priorities focused on the comfort of their positioning and their ability to fulfil lifestyle and functional activities. Carers placed a high priority on the ease of management of the prescribed equipment by a range of different people, and its facility for being transported in a vehicle. Where children were concerned, classroom staff had an expectation that the wheelchair and associated seating would be appropriate for transportation to and within school, and would provide positioning conducive to the working environment.

The approach adopted by the occupational therapist, as clinical lead in this scenario, required a number of skills. She needed to acknowledge the interdependency in achieving a good outcome between:

- the physical needs and prognosis of the disabled person;
- his or her desire to engage with a range of specified meaningful self-care, leisure and productivity activities;
- the person's reliance on carers' contributions in order to facilitate the desired outcomes; and
- the varied personal motivations of carers – for example, paid carers' requirements as part of a job were not the same as a parent's emotional engagement.

The therapist's clinical decision making was supported by her awareness of the service user's disability and the long-term implications of managing this within the environments and networks in which the person lived. This was also informed by her knowledge of the day-to-day handling implications of the equipment and the evident abilities and attitudes of the daily carers. The therapist also required an understanding of the dynamics between the various caregivers, such as parents/partners, classroom assistants and residential home care staff.

Given limited funding budgets and the particular features of the available equipment, the therapist might achieve an outcome that was a relative compromise in provision, but one in which all stakeholders had seen that their particular requirements had been considered. So the best result would be that all involved people would sign up to the use of the new equipment with an understanding that its features were needed by the service user in order to enhance their functional and lifestyle ability, with an additional desire to inhibit a deterioration in condition.

Within such a complex environment, when a large number of stakeholders present views that impact on the therapist's decision making, how does she maintain the service user at centre stage? Should the disabled person's view take precedence, given that his or her life will be influenced in most waking activities by the comfort, support and features of the equipment that they are required to use? Should the carers' needs have a high profile since without daily carer engagement the service user's occupational experiences will be limited? Should the therapist's clinical skills and knowledge and her awareness of likely future deterioration if appropriate postural support is absent take precedence? By revisiting Creek's (2003) definition, it becomes evident that the therapist's global consideration is correct. She has focused on what will be most beneficial to the individual, taking into account the totality of their lived environments and desired activities, including carers' capacities and her own clinical knowledge.

A word on theory

It is important here to consider how an occupational therapist-led clinic in a predominantly biomechanical setting can promote or retain an occupational focus in goal-setting. Hagedorn (1992) reminds us that the therapist applies mechanical principles to the design of assistive technologies following her analysis of movement and functional limitations. The notion of using equipment to enhance functional ability is reinforced by Turner's assertion (Turner et al., 2002) that the compensatory frame of reference supports the provision of external mechanisms in order to compensate for long-term or chronic disorders. Within this theoretical framework, the purpose of special seating is to provide postural support that will save energy and increase functional skills (Ham et al., 1999; Mayall and Desharnais, 1999), thus directly contributing to the individual's ability for participation in chosen activities. The Royal College of Physicians (1995) describes the need for special seating in the following way:

> Some people with poor postural control or fixed skeletal deformity are unable to sit in conventional wheelchairs. Special seating can provide postural control

for these people, enabling retention or promotion of their functional abilities by giving developmentally and biomechanically correct feedback. Correct positioning facilitates improved physical ability and skills. Providing it is supplied early enough, special seating will delay or prevent the onset of deformity by retaining or encouraging the development of symmetrical postures.

(Royal College of Physicians, 1995, p. 18).

Giving consideration to the level of disability experienced by people who require supportive seating, it is evident that many have little or limited motor control due to a range of primarily neurological or genetic disorders, while people with severe learning disabilities may lack the cognitive ability necessary for independent function. The concept of meaningful occupation must therefore include a participatory, experiential or sensory perspective, rather than a focus solely on functional engagement with an activity.

The interview stage

By undertaking individual interviews with a broad range of stakeholders who brought their own agendas and aspirations to the wheelchair clinic, the researcher was able to gain an insight into the priorities and reasoning of each involved person. Thus, the participants were able to weigh up the relative importance of aspects such as mobility provision, user preferences, postural support and psychosocial factors when the prescription of a wheelchair and seating was being considered.

The original 19 subjects were retained in the study for the interview stage, although only 4 of these people had sufficient cognitive ability and communication mechanisms to participate themselves with the interview questions. The remainder were either too young or too impaired to be able to contribute to the study. Additional interviewees included parents and carers (20), occupational therapists (10), physiotherapists (14) and teachers (7). All interviews were undertaken within settings that constituted a regular part of the services user's lifestyle, and included school, home (users' own, parental and residential) and, in one instance to suit the user's occupational pursuit, at a riding school for the disabled. As the interviews took place after the equipment prescribed at the seating clinic had been supplied, an opportunity was available to observe the lived experiences of the service users with the new provisions and to ascertain whether the reality of the outcomes matched the original intentions.

The interviews were highly revealing as the participants, from their hands-on experiences, were considerably better informed about the features, advantages and disadvantages of the equipment than they had been in the exploratory stage of assessment at the seating clinic. They were therefore able to relay quite clearly the aspects they felt should be prioritised when wheelchair and seating provision were being considered.

Although only a small number of participants were the seating users themselves, they were unanimous in their opinion that comfort, postural support to maximise functioning and a pleasing appearance were essential, but they also expressed strong concerns for the welfare of their carers in moving, handling and transporting the equipment. Parents of young children were clear that seating must provide adequate postural support in order to prevent the development of deformities; furthermore, wheelchair seating was only one element in an approach to 24-hours-a-day postural management in which supported lying and standing were also important. A shift of emphasis was apparent as children grew into young people and adults, with increasing parent/carer concern for user comfort, pressure relief, mobility and vehicle transportation needs.

The views of therapists demonstrated professional differences, with physiotherapists focused primarily on postural management and occupational therapists aware of comfort and lifestyle requirements. Teachers unanimously noted the need for adequate postural support to facilitate classroom participation, together with a key need for mobility and manoeuvrability.

Findings, values and implications

The findings of the research provided a fascinating insight into a range of individual values and motivations. Perhaps the most significant finding was the evidence that the provision of a single wheelchair and seating system to an individual provoked an enormous range of perspectives as to its purpose and function. Not only was there some disparity in these perspectives but, more importantly, they were not necessarily identifiable from the assessment process within the clinical setting. Overtly, within the clinic setting, there was a common recognition on the part of healthcare professionals, teaching staff and carers alike that the prescription process for complex wheelchairs and seating systems would result in the supply of equipment that required handling and manoeuvring, but the largely unspoken desire, which became evident from the interviews, was for this to cause as little impact on daily life and routines as possible. Within clinic discussions there was rarely open acknowledgement that the management of pieces of equipment would necessarily incur time and a certain level of physical handling, and would result in some restriction of the freedom of mobility enjoyed by people without impairments. For example, the wheelchair and seating required to fulfil clinical need might not fit inside the family's current vehicle.

Furthermore, there was reluctant acceptance by carers of the inevitability that, as a disabled child grew into a teenager, then an adult, the equipment they required would correspondingly increase in size and weight. The disabled child whose postural and mobility needs might be fulfilled by a buggy which is structurally and aesthetically not very dissimilar to buggies used by other children becomes a young adult whose disability is emphasised by the need for custom-made equipment. Such sensitivities were openly shared with the researcher away from the clinic setting during the interview sessions, where the familiarity of being in a chosen environment and removed from the potentially stressful clinic environment made personal revelations easier.

Maintaining a focus on occupation

When the focus in a clinical setting is on posture, equipment provision and its management, how does the notion of occupation achieve recognition? When working with service users who have such significant disabilities that they may be unable to undertake any activities for themselves, how can the occupational therapist create an environment in which the concept of meaningful occupation becomes a priority in considering the features of seating systems? The findings of the research reported in this chapter provide some response to these questions.

For people whose sitting ability is compromised, having adequate postural management is absolutely essential in order to facilitate any motor functioning and to enable participation in desired activities. By maintaining the use of occupational language within the clinic setting, the occupational therapist can reinforce the overarching reason why optimal postural management is essential: for severely disabled people, adequate postural support enables occupational engagement. The top priority in seating provision expressed by therapists and carers was found to be adequate postural support, and this was reinforced by seating users themselves, whose only higher priority was comfort. By identifying the service user's preferred occupations at an early stage within the assessment process for a wheelchair and seating system, the occupational therapist and other members of the assessment team can ensure that the prescription outcome is designed to facilitate occupational performance – one of the key reasons for providing supportive seating.

Boundaries of therapist reasoning

How often do therapists allow their service users to reason through the options that are available to them when an intervention is planned? Is being client-centred construed as the therapist's perceptions of the service user's needs and wishes obtained through an initial assessment, or does she provide options and insights, assisting the user to reason through and articulate the range of likely outcomes that might be the result of any particular course of action?

Mattingly and Fleming (1994) advise us that:

> Clinical reasoning is a thinking process . . . it involves deliberation about what an appropriate action is in this particular case, with this particular patient, at this particular time.

This perspective reminds the therapist that decisions are made in conjunction with the service user in order to determine an outcome. In practice, options for action are constrained by the circumstances and setting in which the intervention takes place. Therapists are employed to do a job, or work within an organisation's identified brief or mandatory responsibility, and this may be at odds with what their service user would actually like to achieve from the therapeutic intervention. Such boundaries are familiar to occupational therapists, and client-centred practice is always likely to include an implicit caveat 'subject to what can be provided in the circumstances'. While clinical need is an accepted argument for determining funding provision, client preference alone may not be.

Clinical decision making within a complex system

In the complex setting of the wheelchair clinic, the therapist's actions are framed by her knowledge of the service user's diagnosis and likely prognosis, the level of funding available, the features of suitable equipment, the identified lifestyle needs of the service user and the preferences of all stakeholders. The therapist may share consideration of the various features of different wheelchair systems, their advantages, disadvantages and the modifications or accessories that can be supplied, encouraging personal preferences to be expressed in aspects such as colour choice and upholstery options. She can enable some limited access to experiencing handling of the preferred equipment, to ensure that carers are familiar with what can be expected from the new provision. But the final decision of the prescription process is achieved through a combination of clinical knowledge and expertise, informed by the outcome of the assessment process and awareness of equipment availability and service frameworks. The result stems from a combination of identified factors and the outcome is frequently the best compromise in the given circumstances, which aims to fulfil the identified main requirements but may not match all expectations.

The therapist should not regard such a compromise in any way as a weakness or failure on her part. She should resist subsequent requests from care staff, family members or others for repeated alterations to the prescription, to provide an option that might be seen as being smaller, less complicated or a different colour, where she has fulfilled the service user's clinical requirements and provided for occupational needs within the resources available to her. Munday *et al.* (2003), in commenting on complex systems, note:

> [In] social systems, such as health care organizations . . . we can be aware of both our local individual interactions and of the system as a whole. We may attempt to manipulate the system by altering our own interactions but due to its complex nature we cannot control it.
>
> (Munday *et al.*, 2003, pp. 308–9)

In the complex setting of the wheelchair seating clinic, the therapist reaches her clinical decision within the resources that are available to her. She cannot control the wider health, social care and educational agendas that also impact on the outcome of her decisions.

The non-communicant client

One of the key considerations that must be borne in mind when working with people having severe physical or learning disabilities is the individual's ability to communicate. The notion of client-centred practice suggests that the service user is making his or her own contribution to discussions and decision making regarding ongoing therapeutic interventions. But what strategies does the therapist have at her disposal when verbal communication is not an option? It may be possible to elicit a disabled person's views through an alternative communication medium, such as signing, or a regular carer may be closely attuned to the service user's individual mechanism for conveying needs and desires, and be aware of their preferred occupations. In such circumstances, the therapist must adopt an alternative approach for 'listening' to what the service user has to say, and needs to include sufficient time in her schedule to allow the service user to communicate, or to receive information from the relevant carers.

The Mental Capacity Act (Department for Constitutional Affairs, 2005) stresses that when someone does not have the ability to engage in decision making about their treatment then their representative must act in their best interests, based on the beliefs and values that would have been expressed should the person have had the capacity to do so. The research reported in this chapter demonstrates that carers, while presumably well-intentioned, may not give true representation of service users' values as opposed to their own. Whether this is due to a lack of altruism, a lack of insight and awareness or a basic lack of understanding that this is the required role has not been established. Nonetheless, the outcome may be that the therapist's decision making is founded on an advocate's perspective rather than the true values of the individual at the centre of the intervention. Schwartz (2002) advised that the position of advocate attracts privilege based on the presumption of his or her insight into the perceived perceptions of the service user – an insight that the work described here has demonstrated is not always displayed – and that this position of privilege confers some entitlement to participation in clinical decision making.

From the research reported in this chapter, it was identified that service users' views of their preferences and priorities in the provision of assistive technologies were at some variance from those of their healthcare professionals and carers. Many wheelchair seating users have poor verbal communication, and it is customary in a busy clinic setting for a carer's views to be elicited as an alternative. Yet we have seen that carers' agendas can be quite different from those of the person for whom they care and this is something that the therapist must maintain awareness of in her reasoning and decision making.

Conclusion

This chapter has reported on some of the complex aspects that confront an occupational therapist in the setting of a wheelchair and seating clinic, where her service users have a considerable level of disability and depend on a wide range of carers and others who have involvement in their daily lives. By exploring at some depth the values of the individual stakeholders and their expectations from the provision of complex assistive technologies, we have seen that priorities in outcome can vary considerably, creating a challenging situation for the therapist and one in which the end product may not fulfil all expectations of all stakeholders.

The overriding priority for wheelchair seating provision is clinical need. Reflecting on what has been learned from the range of stakeholders it becomes evident that clinical need has several clearly identifiable components in this context – mobility, postural control and prevention of deformity. Ask why any of these components is important and the response is the same: to enable the service user to access, and continue to access, to the best of their abilities the occupations that are important to them.

The key guideline to assist the therapist in her reasoning and actions in a clinic situation is maintaining a focus on the identified clinical need, underpinned by the occupational values of the service user. In situations where a service user is unable to communicate their own occupational needs, the therapist should be clear that a carer advocate is enabled to contribute the service user's known preferences, so that means for fulfilling these can be included.

In reflecting back on the development of this essay, I am drawn again to the findings of Creek's 2003 work. Her analysis of recent occupational therapy literature in the UK describes the elements of occupational therapy practice as: 'therapist, client, context, environment and therapist's actions' (p. 14). The research study described in this chapter very clearly demonstrated all these elements, within a particular occupational therapy-led setting. What our professional literature has, to date, lacked is demonstration of how we bring our unique knowledge, thinking and reasoning skills into this mix. By more overtly using occupational language in our daily practice and reflecting this in our published work, the centrality of occupationally focused interventions as delivered by occupational therapists to the health and well-being of people with disabilities will gain increasing recognition and profile.

References

British Society of Rehabilitation Medicine (1995) *Seating Needs for Complex Disabilities*, British Society of Rehabilitation Medicine, London.

Creek, J. (2003) *Occupational Therapy Defined as a Complex Intervention*, College of Occupational Therapists, London.

Department for Constitutional Affairs (2005) *The Mental Capacity Act*, HMSO, London.

Department of Health (2006) *The National Strategy for Carers* (www.carers.gov.uk/ supportingcarers).

Hagedorn, R. (1992) *Occupational Therapy: Foundations for Practice*, Churchill Livingstone, Edinburgh.

Ham, R., Aldersea, P. and Porter, D. (1999) *Wheelchair Users and Postural Seating: A Clinical Approach*, Churchill Livingstone, Edinburgh.

Mattingly, C. and Fleming, M. (1994) *Clinical Reasoning: Forms of Enquiry in a Therapeutic Practice*, F.A. Davis Co., Philadelphia.

Mayall, J.K. and Desharnais, G. (1999) *Positioning in a Wheelchair*, 2nd edn, Slack, Thorofare, NJ.

Munday, D.F., Johnson, S.A. and Griffiths, F.E. (2003) Complexity theory and palliative care *Palliative Medicine*, **17**, 308–9.

Royal College of Physicians (1995) *The Provision of Wheelchairs and Special Seating: Guidance for Purchasers and Providers*, Royal College of Physicians, London.

Schwartz, L. (2002) Is there an advocate in the house? The role of healthcare professionals in patient advocacy. *Journal of Medical Ethics*, **28**, 37–40.

Turner, A., Foster, M. and Johnson, S.E. (2002) *Occupational Therapy and Physical Dysfunction: Principles, Skulls and Practice*, Churchill Livingstone, Edinburgh.

Engaging the reluctant client

7

Jennifer Creek

Introduction

Activity is one of the main tools used by occupational therapists with their clients to improve and maintain physical and mental health, remediate disability, encourage adaptive behaviour, teach skills and build individual and group identity (Creek, 1998). Activity can be used to promote health and well-being in people experiencing deprivation, developmental delay, disorder and disability (Creek, 2002). However, some of the most needy people can also be the most difficult to engage. Choosing or designing activities to capture the interest and engage the attention of individuals and groups of clients is a core skill of the occupational therapist.

For the occupational therapist, engagement is the experience of involving oneself in an undertaking, occupying oneself in an activity or interest (*New Shorter Oxford English Dictionary*, 1993). Engagement in activity suggests attention and commitment to what is being done, not simply being present in body. When someone is engaged in an activity, his attention is focused on a goal and/or on the experience, not on the skills and effort required. He is absorbed in the activity and pays minimal attention to extraneous thoughts and feelings or to his physical state.

Occupational therapists believe that it is necessary to engage the client in activity rather than simply making sure that he complies with the therapeutic programme. This is because active participation by the individual in the process of therapy, as opposed to passive compliance, increases his choice, autonomy, responsibility for outcomes and control over his care (Creek, 2003). The

American occupational therapist, Peloquin (in Clark *et al.*, 1998, p. 15), suggested that the central role of occupational therapy is 'to engage persons towards the actions that help them build their lives . . . When our therapies fail to engage body, mind, and spirit, our credibility as occupational therapists is at stake.'

This paper explores some of the factors that contribute to the experience of engagement in activity. It begins with a brief discussion of the concept of people as occupational beings, demonstrating that to be human is to be active. However, the degree and nature of activity are influenced by three factors: motivation, volition and autonomy. Each of these concepts is defined and the relationships between them are clarified, showing how they contribute in different ways to engagement. Barriers to engagement are discussed, using illustrations from occupational therapy practice. The final section of the chapter offers suggestions on identifying the barriers for an individual and addressing them.

People as occupational beings

Humans have been described as 'occupational beings' (Wilcock, 1998, p. 3) because we exhibit complex occupational behaviour that 'has allowed us to change, or adapt to and survive healthily, in many different environments'. The American occupational therapist, Mary Reilly (1962, p. 4), described work, in the sense of using one's capacities to alter and control the environment, as 'a physiologically conditioned need and . . . an imperative part of man's nature'. Thirty years later, the occupational scientist, Ann Wilcock (1993), wrote that the need to engage in occupation is innate and is crucial for the maintenance of health and well-being.

Occupational therapists believe that all people share a fundamental drive to be active, to explore and to use one's capacities: indeed, the profession was founded on this belief. Reilly expressed it in this way:

> Man has a vital need for occupation and . . . his central nervous system demands the rich and varied stimuli that solving life's problems provides him and . . . this is the basic need that occupational therapy ought to be serving.
>
> (Reilly, 1962, p. 5)

Sometimes, occupational therapy practitioners forget that activity is the natural state of each person. They talk about people being unmotivated or about the need to motivate clients. This perspective is not compatible with the original philosophy of the profession. For example, Adolph Meyer, a psychiatrist who was involved in the establishment of the profession of occupational therapy in the United States, spoke of activities being used as incentives to encourage acceptable behaviour in patients. The incentive was 'pleasure in achievement, a real pleasure in the use and activity of one's hands and muscles and a happy *appreciation of time*' (Meyer, 1922/1977, p. 640). Dr Elizabeth Casson, who founded the first school of occupational therapy in the United Kingdom, also envisaged occupational therapists working with the human need to be active. She wrote that:

> One of the most powerful motives we have is curiosity. It is so universally active that we often forget it . . . The well-trained occupational therapist uses this active motive in her patients continually . . . Following on the instinct of curiosity comes the desire to achieve. Every child loves to make something that he has made himself.
>
> (Casson, 1935/1955, p. 99)

Each person has an innate need to be active but its expression can be blocked by illness, negative experiences or adverse circumstances, so that the individual can seem disinterested in activity. In order to work out how to engage the client as an active partner in the therapeutic process, especially the reluctant client, the occupational therapist needs to understand three factors:

- The client's drives or *motivation*;
- What influences the choices he makes, that is, his *volition*, and
- The extent to which he is able to think, decide and act for himself, that is, his *autonomy*.

Motivation

Each person has needs that generate the drive to act: for example, the need to eat is experienced as hunger, which directs us to seek food; the need to avoid harm is usually experienced as pain or fear, which causes us to try to escape. This drive to act is called *motivation*, which can be defined as 'the (conscious or unconscious) stimulus, incentive, motives etc. for action towards a goal . . . the factors giving purpose or direction to behaviour' (*New Shorter Oxford English Dictionary*, 1993). The South African occupational therapist, Vona du Toit (1991b), described motivation as the energy source for occupational behaviour and said that it is expressed in action.

Motivation may be extrinsic or intrinsic. Extrinsic motivation is the drive to avoid harm and meet needs, and thus to 'mind the body and maintain health' (Wilcock, 1998, p. 30). It is experienced by the individual as a need to act in response to circumstances. These may be external circumstances, such as the rapid approach of a car, which generates the need to run out of its path. Extrinsic motivation may also be activated by an internal circumstance such as the feeling of hunger, which is experienced as a need to eat. Extrinsic motivators can also be social, such as the needs for approval and belonging.

Intrinsic motivation has been described as 'occurring when an activity satisfies basic human needs for competence and control . . . , which makes the activity interesting and likely to be performed for its own sake rather than as a means to an end' (Sansone and Harackiewicz, 2000, p. 444). Intrinsic motivation is the drive to act for the enjoyment of exercising one's capacities, for learning and for taking pleasure in activity, which Wilcock (1998) described as characteristic of humans as occupational beings. Humans share this basic need to be active with all other living beings, although we express it in more complex and directed ways.

Reilly (1974a) developed a theory of play that takes account of both intrinsic and extrinsic motivation. She described play as a strategy for exploring external reality, processing meanings, understanding what is explored, mastering one's own capacities, finding solutions to problems and adapting to the world. Children naturally choose to engage in play, therefore it must be intrinsically motivated (Reilly, 1974b). Reilly (1974c) proposed that playful behaviour is motivated by the exploratory drive of curiosity, which has three hierarchical stages: exploratory, competency and achievement.

The exploratory stage occurs when an event is new to the individual or different from what has been experienced before. It consists of playful behaviour that is engaged in for its own sake. Exploratory behaviour focuses on sensory experience, and 'in the pure pleasure of doing something for its own sake . . . teases and tests reality as the imagination searches for rules' (Reilly, 1974c, p. 146).

The competency stage is characterised by a drive to deal efficiently with the environment, to have an active influence on it and, in turn, to be influenced by it. Competency behaviour focuses on repeating and practising a task until it is mastered. The critical characteristic of this stage is persistence, which is only elicited if the individual has 'trust in the environment and confidence in self' (Reilly, 1974c, p. 146).

The achievement stage involves measuring the outcomes of behaviour against standards or expectations. Reilly (1974c, p. 147) acknowledged that motivation at this stage has moved from intrinsic to extrinsic because the standard of excellence is linked to external standards of pass/fail, good/bad, win/lose rather than to the individual's private sense of what is acceptable. She suggested that the individual at this stage is focused on performance and is competing with the self or with others. Risk taking and courage are characteristics of this stage.

Using this theory when selecting and adapting an activity to engage the client, the occupational therapist can:

- attract his attention by stimulating his curiosity;
- hold his interest by offering suitable challenges;
- ensure that the activity is relevant to him by matching it to his standards and expectations.

For example, an occupational therapist facilitated a drop-in creative activity group for women living in an area of social and economic deprivation. She made the activities attractive to the women by displaying interesting samples and an exciting variety of materials. Once their interest was captured, she held it by ensuring that the demands of the activity were just beyond the women's capabilities, so that they were always challenged but never overwhelmed. The women valued the end product if it looked as though it had been bought in a shop and/or was valued by other people. The therapist ensured that these standards were met by using high-quality materials and structuring each activity carefully so that the participants were satisfied with what they produced.

An understanding of factors that trigger and maintain motivation can help the occupational therapist to design and select activities that will engage the client, whatever his level of functioning. An understanding of volition allows the therapist to select or adapt activities so that they are at the appropriate level for the client, and to help him to develop further his ability to make choices and engage in voluntary action. The next section of this chapter discusses some of the elements of activity that affect volition and thus influence the degree to which someone might find an activity engaging.

Volition

Each person spends the greater part of his life being active, with variable degrees of intensity depending on his level of motivation, but people do not all do the same activities. The ways in which a person acts, and the activities he chooses, depend on his volition.

Volition is 'the action of consciously willing or resolving something; the making of a definite choice or decision regarding a course of action' (*New Shorter Oxford English Dictionary*, 1993). This definition assumes that volition itself is a mental action. The American philosopher, Ginet (1990, p. 15), said that volition is 'the mental action with which one begins voluntary exertion of the body'. Volition is not a precursor or trigger to action, or a separate action, but is a necessary component of voluntary exertion. It is the awareness, during an activity, of its being performed voluntarily (Creek, 1998). The British philosopher, Ryle (1949/1990), argued that we can say an action is voluntary when a person does something he could have chosen not to do.

When volition is conceptualised as a necessary component of voluntary activity, it can be seen as a skill that can be developed, learned, improved, lost or regained. For occupational therapists, volition can be defined as the skill of being able to perceive and work towards a goal through choosing and performing activities that will achieve desired results.

Some of the factors that affect people's choices of action are:

- interests;
- personal goals and values;
- awareness of our own capacities (Ginsberg *et al.*, 1951);
- the meanings that people give to different activities (Fidler 1999);
- the nature of the choices available;
- knowledge of what activities are available;
- knowledge of how to access different activities;
- capacity to see opportunities for action; and
- having enough information on which to base choices (Creek, 1998).

Interests are the things that arouse a person's curiosity or concern (*New Shorter Oxford English Dictionary*, 1993). For the occupational therapist, they are 'an individual's preferences for occupations based on the experience of pleasure and satisfaction in participating in those activities' (Kielhofner, 1992, p. 157). Personal goals are the individual's desired outcomes or the results that he wants to attain from his actions (Creek, 2003). Personal values are the individual's 'personally held judgement of what is valuable and important in life' (Creek, 2003, p. 60). A person's awareness of his capacities is his ability to predict his own effectiveness in given situations.

The meaning of an activity is the significance or importance that it has for the person performing it (Creek, 1998). People have a fundamental need to understand and give meaning to the experiences and events of their lives and will actively seek meaning in and through activity (Fine, 1999). However, meanings are influenced by the context in which the activity takes place, and meanings change over time. For example, running to catch a bus will have a different meaning from running in order to maintain physical fitness.

The meanings inherent in any activity include both the personal associations that it has for the individual and wider socio-cultural meanings. These two areas of meaning, the personal and the social, are intimately linked. According to the Russian psychologist, Vygotsky, meaning is created through the interaction of the individual with his physical and social world (Newman and Holzman, 1993). Further, Vygotsky claimed that the meaning people give to situations determines which activities they choose to use to achieve their goals.

Activities have both actual and symbolic meanings. A *symbol* is something that represents or recalls something else, 'especially a material object representing an abstract concept or quality' (*New Shorter Oxford English Dictionary*, 1993). For example, an open fire may symbolise warmth and welcome, even in a centrally heated house. The American occupational therapist, Susan Fine (1999), said that the function of symbols is 'connecting the inner life and the consciousness of the individual with the collective belief systems of his or her culture'.

What a person chooses to do is in part dependent on the activities available, both in the short term and the long term. For example, a woman who lives in a small town will not be able to go shopping for clothes in the evening when all the shops are shut. However, she can put off the activity until another day or travel to a shopping centre that has late-night shopping. In order to engage in an activity, a person has to know that the activity can be done, where it can be done and what conditions are necessary to be able to do it. For example, before a man can take a ride in a hot air balloon, he has to be aware that commercial balloon flights are available, he has to know where and how to book such a flight and he has to know how to get to the site.

The capacity to see opportunities for action is linked to having awareness of one's own capacities. For example, if an occupational therapist is looking for a job in primary care, she may find that few such posts are advertised. In order to find the kind of job she wants, she could start by looking at all the jobs being advertised in primary care. For each one, she could take note of the skills and experience being sought, compare them with her own skills and experience and make a judgement about whether or not it is worth her while to apply. In order to make informed choices, it is necessary to have information about the choices available, one's own capacities and the possible outcomes of the different alternatives.

Several of the factors that influence choices of activity are related to the individual's knowledge and abilities; for example, knowing what activities are available and being able to judge one's own capacities. This means that a person's volition, or his ability to make autonomous choices, will vary in different situations. When someone has greater knowledge and understanding of the situation, he is more able to exercise volition. The skill of volition, like any other skill, is learned through experience and practice so that it becomes easier to make choices with practice: the more often someone has opportunities to make decisions about what to do, other circumstances being equal, the more readily he will be able to choose a course of action. Someone who has never had opportunities for making choices or for identifying personal preferences will find it difficult to formulate clear intentions or to make decisions about action. A person who lacks this skill is often said to have a volitional disorder.

So far, an argument has been made for differentiating between the concepts of motivation and volition. Motivation is defined as the basic drive to be active that is shared by everyone, while volition is the skill of being able to make autonomous choices and decisions about what action to take. The third factor to consider when engaging the client in activity is autonomy.

Autonomy

Autonomy is 'the capacity to think, decide, and act on the basis of such thought and decision freely and independently and without . . . let or hindrance' (Gillon 1985, 1986, p. 60). A person may have a high level of motivation and good volitional ability, but his autonomy can still be compromised by the circumstances in which he finds himself. For example, an occupational therapist feels strongly enough about a professional issue to want to share her opinion with others (motivation). She chooses to write an opinion piece for her professional journal and plans exactly what she will say (volition). Then a colleague takes sick leave and the service manager decides that all the other therapists in the department must give up their continuing professional development time in order to provide cover (autonomy). The therapist wants to open a debate on an important issue and knows what to do about it, but she does not have the time to take action.

The moral philosopher, Gillon (1985, 1986), suggested that the ability to make and enact choices rests on three types of autonomy:

- autonomy of thought: being able to think for oneself, to have preferences and to make decisions;
- autonomy of will: having the freedom to decide to do things on the basis of one's deliberations;
- autonomy of action: the capacity to act on the basis of reasoning.

The therapist described above is able to think for herself and have an opinion about the issue that is concerning her: she has autonomy of thought. She is able to decide to write a paper in order to share her concerns: she has autonomy of will. But she is not able to find time to write because of lack of resources at work: she does not, on this occasion, have autonomy of action.

Autonomy is not an all-or-nothing condition but varies for the same person at different times: on another occasion, the therapist may apply for study leave to work on a project and be given the time she needs. Not only does an individual's level of autonomy fluctuate, but different people have varying levels of autonomy. For example, a woman who has always lived alone will be accustomed to making decisions for herself on a daily basis. A woman who has been in a close relationship for most of her life will find it difficult at first to make independent decisions if she loses her partner.

Conditions that may affect someone's autonomy include:

- personal circumstances: for example, an individual's choice of activities may be limited by temporary or permanent bodily impairment;
- environmental barriers: for example, it is not possible to go ice-skating unless there is access to ice;
- social pressures: for example, a boy living in an urban environment in the north-east of England might be reluctant to take ballet lessons because of fear that his peers would mock him.

The Chilean economist, Max Neef, and colleagues suggested that autonomy can be compromised by external factors, such as constraint, oppression or lack of resources, or by internal factors, such as fear, ignorance or passivity (Max Neef *et al.*, 1991). An example of external constraints limiting autonomy is the occupational therapist, working single-handedly within a community mental health team, who finds herself unable to keep occupation at the centre of her practice because of pressure from colleagues to share the generic work of the team. An example of internal factors limiting autonomy is the occupational therapist who would like to work on a freelance basis but is afraid of failing and so stays in a job that she does not find fulfilling.

When a person performs an activity voluntarily, there is an interplay between motivation, volition and autonomy that determines which activity he chooses and the extent to which he becomes engaged in what he is doing. Problems with motivation, volition or autonomy can interfere with an individual's ability to initiate or commit to action. The next section explores how the occupational therapist might identify the reasons why a client is reluctant to participate in therapeutic activity, thus enabling her to modify her approach.

The reluctant client

In order to reach therapeutic goals, the therapist works with the client to select activities that will meet his needs, develop his skills and engage his interest. However, when the therapist invites a client to join in an activity, there is always the possibility that he will refuse. There may be several reasons for this:

- The client has a problem with motivation and cannot find sufficient energy to participate in this particular activity at this time;
- The client has a volitional disorder that prevents him from initiating action or insufficient information to enable him to choose to participate;

- The client is blocked from participating because his autonomy is compromised by internal or external circumstances;
- The client has thought rationally about the activity and his decision not to participate is a reasonable one.

If the client's level of motivation is low, he may feel too fatigued to do the activity that the therapist is suggesting. This is common, for example, if someone is severely depressed. In this case, the therapist either waits until the client is feeling more energetic or finds an activity that is within his present capabilities. It might be possible to do a one-to-one session with the client, making a cup of tea rather than expecting him to work with several other people to cook a meal. It is important to make the activity attractive to the client and, if possible, trigger his curiosity motivation. Once the client attempts the activity, the therapist provides encouragement and support so that he is able to reach his optimum activity level. If the client is severely depressed, the first few sessions may be spent sitting with him and making undemanding conversation until he feels ready to do something more active.

The second possibility is that the client is having difficulty choosing whether or not to participate. Giving more information about the activity, in a form that the client can understand, may be all that is needed to overcome the problem. However, it may be that the client has a volitional disorder that is interfering with his capacity to make choices. Perhaps he has never tried cooking and does not know if he would enjoy it. Or perhaps he lacks self-confidence and is afraid of failing in front of other people. If the problem seems to be one of volition, the therapist can help the client to develop this skill by giving him opportunities to have new experiences, starting with undemanding activities and giving enough support so that he experiences success. Enough time has to be allowed for the client to practise any new activity until he feels confident about doing it and happy with the standard he has reached.

The third possibility is that the client is not able to make the choice to participate freely and independently because his autonomy is compromised. For example, he may be experiencing auditory hallucinations that are interfering with his ability to concentrate. In this case, the therapist can help the client to identify what is preventing him from making his own decisions, or acting on the basis of his decisions, and work with him to find ways of overcoming those barriers.

Within the controlled conditions of an occupational therapy session, it is possible to ensure that suitable conditions are in place to enable the client to choose activities that he wants to do and to support him in carrying them out. Outside the therapeutic situation, the client may encounter a range of physical, economic or social barriers to action. It is part of the occupational therapist's role to help the client to identify these obstacles and to find ways round them, thus increasing his capacity for autonomous action.

When a client does not want to join in an activity, there is also the possibility that this is an autonomous decision. If the client could do the activity but is choosing not to, freely and independently, in full knowledge of what the activity would entail and what missing it means, then the therapist can assume that this is a reasonable decision. Perhaps the client knows how to cook but does not enjoy it, or perhaps he is expecting a visitor at the time when the cookery group is meeting. If the therapist is satisfied that the client's decision not to do the activity is an autonomous one, then it is important to respect that choice, thus supporting the client's autonomy.

The occupational therapist using a person-centred approach will take time to identify with the client those activities that have the potential not only to bring about positive change but also to attract and hold the client's attention and interest. To find the most appropriate activities for a particular individual, the therapist has to take into account the nature of both the client and the activity. She considers the client's motivational level, personal choices and autonomy. In addition, she analyses activities for the elements that might promote or inhibit engagement. In this way, she can find the best fit between the client, the activity and the requirement to reach therapeutic goals.

Factors that promote or inhibit engagement

Analysis and reflection are two types of thinking that can assist the occupational therapist to select or adapt activities in order to promote engagement for individuals and groups of clients. Activity analysis enables the therapist to identify the properties of the activity, while reflection promotes understanding of how people might respond to and interact with those properties.

Analysis is a mode of thinking used to break a complex phenomenon into its simple elements (*New Shorter Oxford English Dictionary*, 1993). Activity analysis is 'a process of dissecting an activity into its component parts and task sequence in order to identify its inherent properties and the skills required for its performance, thus allowing the therapist to evaluate its therapeutic potential' (Creek, 2003, p. 49). The occupational therapist analyses activities in order to identify 'all the effects that activities can potentially provide, simultaneously and sequentially' (Breines, 1995, p. 26).

In addition to activity analysis, the therapist uses another mode of thinking in order to try to understand the experience of activity: reflection. Reflection is a mode of thinking 'in which people recapture their experience, think about it, mull it over and evaluate it' (Boud *et al.*, 1985, in Kember *et al.*, 2001, p. 21). It is subjective, seeking to understand the personal experience of an individual doing an activity on a particular occasion, rather than looking for those elements that can be observed objectively or analysed logically. The American occupational therapist, Betty Hasselkus (2002, p. 8), described how people 'weigh their experiences and expectations and thereby construct personal meanings of events and phenomena'.

Activity analysis and reflection can be used to identify those elements of an activity that have the potential to affect the participant's level of engagement by influencing his motivation, volition and autonomy. These elements may be:

- aspects of the activity;
- characteristics of the person performing the activity; or
- features of the social and cultural context of the activity.

Elements inherent in the activity that have the potential to influence engagement include, for example, the amount of physical effort required, how messy the activity is, and the opportunities it offers for having an effect on the environment or for learning new skills. All activities involve some degree of discipline and have, within their materials, equipment, environment, rules and process, inherent frustrations, limitations, constraints or coercion. For example, a game of football has a single ball of a particular type, the same number of players on each side, a pitch with features such as goals and a centre, rules about where players can go and how they can interact and a process for playing the game. Whether the game is a professional league match or a spontaneous knock-about in the park, all these features will be present to some extent and will guide and constrain how participants can act.

The therapist can identify the features inherent in the activity by doing it herself and then analysing the conditions and demands that it imposes. She can become aware of her own responses to these conditions and demands by reflecting on the experience of activity. Deeper reflection leads to a more comprehensive understanding of why we react to particular conditions in certain ways. For example, a therapist might come to realise that she avoids doing messy activities, such as pottery, with her clients. A longer period of reflection on this brings up a memory of her mother getting anxious whenever anything was spilled or otherwise out of order in the house. Without the therapist being consciously aware of it, she has been responding still to her mother's anxiety by trying to avoid making a mess.

Such personal reflections reveal the therapist's responses to activity and can increase her sensitivity to the very different reactions that clients might have to the same activity. However, it is only possible to elicit the client's memories, associations and meanings by taking time to observe and listen to his version of what is happening. The personal dimension of engagement in activity means that it is not always possible to predict precisely how a client will respond to an activity, especially if the person has had limited life experiences and is not able to tell the therapist what he enjoys or does not enjoy doing. Sometimes, it is necessary to try out a few activities with the client so that he can experience and reflect on how he feels about them.

Hasselkus (2002) emphasised the importance of recognising that the therapist and client will have different perceptions of the same events, or different stories. She described 'a therapeutic approach that incorporates time and strategies to gain understanding of the client's history and story and to share the therapist's story with the client' (p. 9). This does not mean sharing the therapist's personal story but how she 'interprets the events and experiences that the therapist and client will create as they weave a new story together' (Hasselkus, 2002, p. 8).

The American anthropologist, Cheryl Mattingly (1994), said that, in each therapeutic encounter, the therapist must ask herself, what story am I in? She described how stories help the therapist to frame practical decisions about what to do, through imposing a narrative structure on the situation. Stories have alternative endings and the therapist and client together can select the ending they want to work towards.

Some elements that influence engagement in activity arise from the social and cultural context in which the activity is being performed. These include, for example, the purpose of the activity, the symbolism of the materials and processes used, the age and sex appropriateness of the activity and the value it is given. The same activity can have very different meanings and value in different cultures. For example, in a crowded city such as Hong Kong, inviting friends to dinner usually means taking them to a restaurant, while having friends to dinner in the UK usually means cooking for them in the home.

When the therapist is thinking about which activity to use with a client, or group of clients, she needs to be sensitive to the possibility of different cultural interpretations of what is being done. If a client reacts in an unexpected way to the activity, it may be that he understands it in a different way from the therapist. For example, a British therapist teaching in the Netherlands asked her students to make Christmas cards, thinking that this was an appropriate activity for the time of year. She was told that home-made cards were not valued within the culture so that the students thought the activity was a waste of time.

As the therapist gains awareness of the many attributes of activity and of different activities, and develops sensitivity to the ways in which people experience and interpret activity, she learns how to select, adapt and facilitate activities to engage even the most reluctant client.

Summary

This essay has argued that occupational therapy is most effective when the client is actively engaged in the therapeutic process rather than being a passive recipient of professional expertise. This active involvement allows the client not simply to comply with a programme to remediate dysfunction but to build or rebuild his own life. However, some of the people who have the greatest need of such individualised therapy have problems that make it difficult for them to engage in partnership working with the therapist.

One of the essential skills of the occupational therapist is being able to overcome barriers and engage the client in therapy. When faced with a reluctant client, the therapist needs to consider three factors that influence engagement: motivation, volition and autonomy. Motivation is conceptualised as the energy source for action, volition is the skill of being able to make choices and autonomy is a condition for the expression of volition.

The skilled therapist is able to identify the client's level of motivation and select appropriate activities. She provides opportunities for the client to develop and practise volition. Finally, she helps him to identify barriers to autonomy and find ways of overcoming them. In this way, the occupational therapist enables clients to achieve the natural state of active participation in the world.

References

Breines, E.B. (1995) Occupational Therapy Activities from Clay to Computers: Theory and Practice, F.A. Davis Co., Philadelphia.

Casson, E. (1935/1955) Occupational therapy. Occupational Therapy, **18**(3), 98–100 (reprinted from Report of the Conference on Welfare of Cripples and Invalid Children, November 1935).

Clark, F., Wood, W. and Larson, E.A. (1998) Occupational science: occupational therapy's legacy for the 21st century, in Willard and Spackman's Occupational Therapy, 9th edn (eds M.E. Neistadt and E.B. Crepeau), Lippincott, Philadelphia, pp. 13–21.

Creek, J. (1998) Purposeful activity, in Occupational Therapy: New Perspectives (ed. J. Creek), Whurr Publishers Ltd, London, pp. 16–28.

Creek, J. (2002) Treatment planning and implementation, in Occupational Therapy and Mental Health, 3rd edn (ed. J. Creek), Churchill Livingstone, Edinburgh, pp. 119–38.

Creek, J. (2003) Occupational Therapy Defined as a Complex Intervention, College of Occupational Therapists, London.

Du Toit, V. (1991a) Creative ability, in Patient Volition and Action in Occupational Therapy 2nd edition (V. du Toit), Vona and Marie du Toit Foundation, Hillbrow, South Africa, pp. 21–35.

Du Toit, V. (1991b) The background theory related to creative ability which leads to work capacity within the context of occupational therapy for the cerebral palsied, in *Patient Volition and Action in Occupational Therapy 2nd edition* (V. du Toit), Vona and Marie du Toit Foundation, Hillbrow, South Africa, pp. 47–54.

Fidler, G.S. (1999) Exploring potential: the activity laboratory, in *Activities: Reality and Symbol* (eds G.S. Fidler and B.P. Velde), Slack, Thorofare, NJ, pp. 27–34.

Fine, S.B. (1999) Symbolization: making meaning for self and society, in *Activities: Reality and Symbol* (eds G.S. Fidler and B.P. Velde), Slack, Thorofare, NJ, pp. 11–25.

Gillon, R. (1985/1986) *Philosophical Medical Ethics*, John Wiley & Sons, Chichester, UK.

Ginet, C. (1990) *On Action*, Cambridge University Press, Cambridge, UK.

Ginsberg, E., Ginsberg, S.W., Axelrad, S. and Herma, J.L. (1951) *Occupational Choice: An Approach to a General Theory*, Columbia University Press, New York.

Hasselkus, B.R. (2002) *The Meaning of Everyday Occupation*, Slack, Thorofare, NJ.

Kember, D., Wong, F.K.Y. and Yeung, E. (2001) The nature of reflection, in *Reflective Teaching and Learning in the Health Professions* (ed. D. Kember), Blackwell, Oxford, UK, pp. 3–28.

Kielhofner, G. (1992) *Conceptual Foundations of Occupational Therapy*, F.A. Davis Co., Philadelphia.

Mattingly, C. (1994) The narrative nature of clinical reasoning, in *Clinical Reasoning: Forms of Inquiry in a Therapeutic Practice* (eds C. Mattingly and M.H. Fleming), F.A. Davis Co., Philadelphia, pp. 239–69.

Max Neef, M.A., Elizalde, A. and Hopenhayn, M. (1991) Development and human needs, in *Human Scale Development: Conception, Application and Further Reflections* (M.A. Max Neef), Apex, New York and London, pp. 13–54.

Meyer, A. (1977) The philosophy of occupation therapy *American Journal of Occupational Therapy*, **31**(10), 639–42 (reprinted from *Archives of Occupational Therapy* (1922), **1**, 1–10).

New Shorter Oxford English Dictionary (1993) Clarendon Press, Oxford.

Newman, F. and Holzman, L. (1993) *Lev Vygotsky: Revolutionary Scientist*, Routledge, London and New York.

Reilly, M. (1962) Occupational therapy can be one of the great ideas of 20th century medicine. *American Journal of Occupational Therapy*, **16**(1), 1–9.

Reilly, M (1974a) Introduction, in *Play as Exploratory Learning* (ed. M. Reilly), Sage Publications, Beverley Hills, CA.

Reilly, M. (1974b) Defining a cobweb, in *Play as Exploratory Learning* (ed. M. Reilly), Sage Publications, Beverley Hills, CA.

Reilly, M. (1974c) An explanation of play, in *Play as Exploratory Learning* (ed. M. Reilly), Sage Publications, Beverley Hills, CA.

Ryle, G. (1949/1990) *The Concept of Mind*, Penguin, Harmondsworth, UK.

Sansone, C. and Harackiewicz, J.M. (2000) Controversies and new directions – is it déjà vu all over again? in *Intrinsic and Extrinsic Motivation: The Search for Optimal*

Motivation and Performance (eds C. Sansone and J.M. Harackiewicz), Academic Press, San Diego, CA.

Schön, D.A. (1983) *The Reflective Practitioner: How Professionals Think in Action*, Basic Books, New York.

Wilcock, A. (1993) A theory of the human need for occupation. *Occupational Science: Australia*, **1**(1), 1–8.

Wilcock, A. (1998) A theory of occupation and health, in *Occupational Therapy: New Perspectives* (ed. J. Creek), Whurr Publishers Ltd, London.

Exploring the facets of clinical reasoning

8

Kit Sinclair

Introduction

All health care professionals work with patients whose problems are character-ised as being complex, unique and often ambiguous. Clinical reasoning is described as the thought processes used by health care professionals to address these prob-lems. The goal of clinical reasoning is wise action based on best judgement in a specific context (Jones, 1997). Concepts related to clinical reasoning can be viewed as descriptors of mental processes that become proficient through clinical experience (Benner, 1984; Dreyfus and Dreyfus, 1986). They can also be viewed as a thinking frame, a structure to organise and support clinical thinking (Perkins, 1987).

In an attempt to discover new perspectives on clinical reasoning and teaching for improved clinical reasoning, an action research project was undertaken in Hong Kong. Part of this project involved the interviewing of twelve occupational therapists directly after a patient interaction. The interviews were analysed to identify components of clinical reasoning which support the actions undertaken by therapists when working with their patients.

Literature review

A seminal study of clinical reasoning in occupational therapy was undertaken in the early 1980s to gain a broader understanding of how therapists make sense of clinical situations and how they decide on the progress of therapy. The American

Occupational Therapy Foundation completed the AOTF Clinical Reasoning Study in 1988. Fleming (1991) reported from this study that experienced therapists utilise three tracks of reasoning called procedural, interactive and conditional tracks. She noted that these three tracks were intertwined. Types, styles and process of reasoning subsequently became a topic of much discussion in the occupational therapy literature (Crabtree, 1998; Schell and Cervero, 1993).

Theorists have attempted to research and further explain clinical reasoning in the occupational therapy literature using descriptors of procedural, theoretical, interactive, diagnostic, scientific, pragmatic, narrative, ethical and conditional reasoning (Schell and Cervero, 1993). These various strategies are used throughout the occupational therapy process and can be related to various facets identified in this research and which contribute to the resulting matrix of clinical reasoning.

Development of competence

Development of skills over time has been studied in a variety of professions to determine the aspects which characterise increasing competence to carry out professionally related activities. Dreyfus and Dreyfus (1986) identified five stages in the skill acquisition model of development of competence from novice to expert. They noted that, with increasing competence, practitioners progressively depart from a reliance on abstract principles and increasingly rely on past, concrete experiences to guide actions. Different levels of competence are characterised by qualitatively different perceptions of tasks, situations and modes of decision making. The situation is seen increasingly as a complex whole within which only certain elements are relevant at a particular time. The development of clinical reasoning follows a stage model showing changed perceptions of the task environment and mode of behaviour. As described by Benner (1984), the development of levels extends from the novices' reasoning based on a highly structured 'cookbook' process involving visual cues and strict adherence to protocols and guidelines, and extends on to the expert therapist's ability to use intuitive thinking to develop goals based on patients' needs. Table 8.1 briefly describes the stages.

In order to view the progressive development of skill and competence over time, these ideas were incorporated into the research undertaken.

Methodology

The sample consisted of 12 occupational therapists working in a variety of clinical settings in the Hong Kong Hospital Authority, a quasi-governmental organisation. The sampling had a purposive perspective, statistically drawn from the total

Table 8.1 Stages of skill acquisition

Stage	Description
Novice	Dependent on theory to guide practice
Advanced beginner	Still procedural but recognises patterns of behaviour
Competent	Able to use both situational thinking and prioritising of concerns. Procedural aspects are more automated
Proficient	Putting it all together
Expert	Quick and intuitive. Able to criticise and re-evaluate decisions

Source: adapted from Dreyfus and Dreyfus (1986) and Benner (1984)

800 occupational therapists in Hong Kong, with a view to gaining a sample from a variety of clinical fields and from therapists with a variety of years of experience. Ethical consent was gained from the hospital research committees for the study. Consent forms were signed by all therapists and patients involved in the study.

The data included transcripts of therapist–patient interaction, transcripts of interview with therapist immediately after the therapy session, and field notes of the interviewer.

The purpose of the study was to note differences and similarities in the clinical reasoning undertaken by occupational therapists working in different fields. The experience of the sample of twelve therapists ranged from 2 to over 15 years. As the main purpose was to explore and identify components of clinical reasoning, the research did not emphasise years of experience, but rather the quality of the specific experience of the therapist at the point of interview. Neither was the purpose to judge the overall performance ability of the therapist.

Transcripts of the recorded therapy session were analysed to gain a sense of general interaction and process, reviewing the therapist's use of protocol, planning and flexibility in thinking. Therapists' interview data was then analysed to identify rationale for data gathering and actions, explanations of tools used or not used, identification of key concepts, depth of judgement and consideration of ramifications of actions. An overall analysis of the session initially placed therapists on a scale of 'novice' to 'expert'.

Table 8.2 Facets identified through analysis of therapists' data

Facets identified	Including
Evidence discovery	recognising clinical cues and defining patient problems
Theory application	personal theory and formal theory
Decision making	identifying what disease and disability mean to the patient, anticipating the patient's future, and the treatment process as storytelling and story creation
Judgement	reflective judgement, rationalising and justifying decisions
Ethics	justifying treatment approaches, pragmatic considerations in treatment, patient-centred reasoning, and therapist's beliefs and personal schema

The constant comparative method was used for analysing the data from therapists with reference to the literature. In correlating these findings to the occupational therapy and health care literature, connections were noted and theoretical foundations incorporated. By moving back and forth between data analysis and reading, a matrix was refined to make sense of the data content. From the process, the researcher identified facets of reasoning important to the occupational therapy process and implicit in reasoning, including evidence discovery, theory application, decision making, judgement and ethics (see Table 8.2). The Sinclair Matrix is a product of this process (see Table 8.3, pages 148–9).

Facets of clinical reasoning in occupational therapy which were identified were then used to further elucidate the level of reasoning of the therapists. The facets are described here in some detail.

Evidence discovery

Evidence discovery includes evidence seeking and data gathering. This involves the aspects of problem sensing, cue recognition and problem definition.

Problem sensing

Problem sensing is establishing what problems might be identified for a patient (Bridge and Twible, 1997). Data must be identified from various perspectives including the objective and subjective data, the historical and current data. Objective data refers to the facts usually established through objective assessment. Subjective data refers to that which is opinion, what the patient or family members think about the situation.

Cue recognition

Underpinning all dimensions of clinical reasoning is the ability of the therapist to recognise relevant clinical cues (evidence discovery) and their relationship to other cues and test or verify them through further examination. Cues are environmental triggers or prompts to memory that guide memory search and are influenced by attention, vigilance and management (Boshuizen and Schmidt, 1995; Dutton, 1995). They exist in the behavioural, psychosocial, cultural and contextual aspects of the patient's situation (Bridge and Twible, 1997).

Problem definition

Patients' problems are defined by therapists based on cues gathered from the results of the assessments. Problems identified are directed to the patient's disabilities, thus linking the patient's problems to the intervention process – that is, applying the tools and procedures of occupational therapy to the issues or problems identified. It is the process needed to create a plan of intervention, implement the plan, and determine when to end or revise the implementation (Reed and Sanderson, 1999). This type of thinking taps the therapist's knowledge about specific diseases and their affect on function (Fleming, 1991). It combines evidence discovery with theory application and basic decision making. It is a more linear process that may be used by the beginner or by a therapist who is unfamiliar with the clinical area as it provides the structure for decision making about probable problems and causes, sometimes referred to as procedural reasoning.

Theory application

It is suggested that theory gives direction for thinking, information about alternatives, and expectations of function and deficits (Mattingly and Fleming, 1994). Though clinical reasoning has a foundation in the therapist's scientific knowledge about disease, human functioning and human occupation, sometimes referred to as formal theory, theoretical knowledge in itself is insufficient for effective clinical reasoning (Higgs et al., 2004). In the presence of ill-defined problems or situations, therapists must make decisions often based on their own practical, tacit

Table 8.3 Sinclair Matrix of Clinical Reasoning

	Novice	Advanced beginner	Competent	Proficient	Expert
Evidence discovery Problem sensing, formulation and definition	May be distracted by irrelevant information. Not able to sort evidence, not looking for evidence.	Seeking evidence, facts or knowledge by identifying relevant sources.	Gathers objective, subjective, historical and current data in organized manner. Distinguishes essential from non-essential data.	Obtains data from all sources. Verifies relevant information. Identifies logical inconsistencies or fallacies. Interprets data back to client.	Diligent and focused in inquiry– takes new evidence and applies it to current situations. Clear understanding of issues. Recognises multiple perspectives. Identifies missing data. Questions the accepted.
Theory application Knowledge and concept development	Dependent on theory to guide thinking. Objective attributes recognised without situational experience such as objective measurable parameters. Limited and inflexible context-free application of rules.	Incorporates contextual information into rule-based thinking. Recognises differences between theoretical expectations and presenting problems (but unable to respond to situation quickly).	Relating theoretical concept (condition, nature, form or function) to context. Interprets data using relevant theoretical constructs.	Combines different diagnostic and procedural approaches with flexibility and creativity. Putting it all together. No longer relies on guidelines to direct appropriate action for situation. Recognises assumptions.	Cognitive reasoning is quick and intuitive with solutions to ill-structured problems. Can predict multiple outcomes. Engages global view and applies theory in a global way. Recognizes meaningful patterns and determines generalisations.
Decision making Evaluating, planning, prioritising, predicting	Uses rule-based procedural reasoning to guide 'actions' but doesn't recognise cues and therefore is not	Still procedural, but can recognise some patterns of behaviour or symptoms, so doesn't prioritise	Procedural aspects more automatic and organised, so able to prioritise problems and plan deliberately, efficiently, and in	Perceives situations as wholes, can anticipate situation and avoid irrelevant information. Prioritise issues (in	Shows confidence in own reasoning abilities: schema based, automated processing. Rapid, methodical, and critical evaluations of solutions. Takes nothing for granted. Meets

Treatment approach	skilful in adapting rules to fit situation. Responds to every need and request with almost equal intensity and speed (not able to prioritise).	data well or identify what is most important.	response to urgency and contextual issues (including background, relationships and environment, relevant to situation). Can see actions in terms of long-range goals. Selects tactics pragmatically.	HK style). Predicts multiple outcomes. Evaluates action, recognizes relationship of action and inaction. Supervisory responsibilities. Liaises with outside organisations for benefit of others.	multiple patient requests and care needs or crisis management without losing important information or missing significant needs. Prioritises quickly and efficiently. Mentors others in decision making skills.
Judgment Including reflective judgement	Unable to use discriminatory judgement. Unreflective—informed by routine. Unable to deal with unfamiliar situations.	Unable to determine priorities, makes judgement based on established criteria/rules. Reflective only after the event, if at all.	Drawing inferences or conclusions that are supported or justified by evidence. Professional autonomy in decision making. Conscious deliberation.	Receptive to divergent views and sensitive to own biases. Recognises ramifications of actions.	Shows confidence in own reasoning abilities. Applies judgement prudently in relevant context, integrates feedback from others to improve practice. Insight into societal conditions generating a patient's illness.
Ethics Including client orientation and documentation	Recognises overt ethical issues. Defends views based on preconceptions.	Begins to recognise more subtle ethical issues, judging according to established personal, professional or social rules or criteria.	Recognises ethical dilemmas. Recognises individual differences. Sensitive to client's views. Contextual considerations. Equality of practice—same rules for all.	More sophisticated in recognising situational nature of ethical reasoning. Provides options, explains outcomes, outlines time sequences for client.	Demonstrates clear understanding of ethical issues and practices ethically, uses practical wisdom. Honest in facing personal bias. Evaluates soundness of conclusions and worth of action to client and others.

knowledge. This is sometimes observed as a personal theory of how to deal with occurrences in the therapy situation (Chapparo and Ranka, 2000).

Formal theory

Formal theory is that which is learned through education, study and reading (Smith, 1992). A person develops formal theories by reading books and testing personal thinking against ideas found there, by reviewing concepts and coming to terms with them. These theories must be examined with the view to developing a defensible personal theory of professional practice.

Personal theory

Personal theory or espoused theory is described by Argyris and Schön (1974) to denote theory which we say we hold and which we believe should direct our actions. In order to use theory appropriately, therapists need to be alert to the messy and complex nature of practice and treat the knowledge that one has as adaptable.

The combination of formal theory and personal theory support the practical implementation of everyday practice in the context of the specific situation as it presents itself. Higgs et al. (2004) suggest that practice knowledge operates as an interconnection of the therapist's discipline, culture and society. Carr notes that 'understanding and applying principles are not . . . two separate processes but mutually constitutive elements in the continuous dialectical reconstruction or transformation of knowledge and action' (Carr, 1995, p. 69). This may be referred to as 'theorizing practice' (Fish and Coles, 1998).

Practice cannot always be theory-guided (Carr, 1995) as practice involves actions for which there may be no direct theory to apply. It is similarly impossible to quote theory for every specific action we make in practice. This may lead to the supposition that we will never establish practice that is totally evidence based, as seems to be the desired trend at the moment in health care.

Decision making

Decision making in occupational therapy involves evaluating, planning, prioritis-ing and predicting. It includes problem-solving strategies such as identifying what disease and disability mean to the patient, anticipating the patient's future and justifying treatment approaches.

At the most basic level, reasoning and decision making are guided by personal values and beliefs that have been acquired over time and reflect the physical, cultural and social environment in which development occurs (Bridge and Twible,

1997). They rely on prior experience and reference to similar cases or lessons learned in that context, which have been stored in memory.

Understanding of the patient is fundamental to the treatment process. This includes the patient's needs, goals, lifestyle, and personal and cultural values. The therapist must have knowledge of the patient's abilities and deficits, as well as insight into motivations and long-term potential.

Identifying what disease and disability mean to the patient

Therapists must understand the patient as a person, not just in relation to disability but also in relation to that person's environment and culture (evidence discovery). This strategy for understanding has been identified in the literature as interactive reasoning (Fleming, 1991). It yields an understanding of what the disease or disability means to the patient (patient's illness experience) (Neistadt *et al.*, 1998). It also encompasses the interpersonal interaction between the therapist and patient (Fleming, 1991; Schwartzberg, 2002) which allows the patient to share the experience of disability and subjective feelings about the treatment they receive. Therapists are thus better able to address the patient's specific needs and preferences with appropriate treatment (Alnervik and Sviden, 1996; Fortmeier and Thanning, 2002).

Anticipating the patient's future

Therapists must revise treatment moment to moment to meet a patient's needs (Neistadt *et al.*, 1998). This revision is done with an eye to the patient's current and possible future contexts. It requires the therapists' ability to understand and see patients as they see themselves and the ability to project a picture for a person's future. It attempts to understand the impact of disability in the context of a patient's life (Mattingly and Fleming, 1994, p. 197) and to anticipate the way in which the condition will affect progress of treatment, the course of treatment and effect of residual disability on future life. Crabtree (1998) describes this as conditional reasoning, a condensing of information into a meaningful whole, like the gestalt of therapy, the whole picture encompassing other processes of reasoning which break down the complexities of therapy into manageable parts, each serving to focus therapy in some way.

Justifying treatment approaches

The part of clinical reasoning associated with a therapist's ability to present a rationale for the chosen treatment approach has been described as scientific reasoning (Hooper, 1997; Rogers, 1983, 1986; Schell and Cervero, 1993). Crabtree (1998) suggests it is a problem-solving image of clinical reasoning based on logic which is highly valued by funding agencies because it appears to offer 'proof' of effectiveness. It involves selecting or changing a treatment approach and understanding why a treatment approach may produce a certain result, based on the assumption that a cause-and-effect relationship exists in most treatment strategies.

This aspect of decision making articulates the conceptual theories for why the treatment is considered effective (evidence-based practice). It uses applied science or applied theory characteristic of the medical profession as a method of framing clinical problems. It is essential to practice, but may be insufficient for many clinical situations (Schell and Cervero, 1993).

The treatment process as story telling and story creation

Therapists reason narratively when they are concerned with disability as an illness experience, that is, with how a physiological condition is affecting the person's life (Fortmeier and Thanning, 2002). Narrative reasoning (Mattingly, 1991) is described as the means of reflecting on past clinical events as well as shaping future treatment decisions, of 'storytelling' and 'story creation'. It is concerned more with the patient's experience of a diagnosis than the diagnosis itself. It yields the patient's occupational history, for example his life history as told through preferred activities, habits and roles.

Judgement

Judgement is the ability to draw inferences and conclusions supported and justified by the use of evidence. It articulates the conceptual theories for why the intervention is considered effective (evidence-based practice) and is based in the reflective judgement epistemology of King and Kitchner (1985). This reflective judgement perspective is an essential part of clinical reasoning, bringing in the personal ability to weigh arguments and make 'best' decisions. Judgement involves recognising the ramifications of decisions and actions and taking responsibility for decisions made.

Therapists must be able to justify treatment based on criteria such as weight of evidence, utility of solutions, and pragmatic need for action. They need to reflect on their actions to improve skills. Therapists must be receptive to divergent views;

not just considering their own version of events, but weighing up all aspects of an issue. Effective communication and justification of clinical decisions to members of the health team, as well as the client and family, are essential to the development of this facet. It is important to provide a clear and credible explanation of the scientific and therapeutic basis for actions in the context of the client's needs and situation.

Ethics

Ethical reasoning encompasses awareness of issues, sensitivity to how one affects other people, willingness to try to overcome obstacles by making best decisions, and the ability and motivation to implement 'best' solutions. This motivation acknowledges that 'moral values are often in competition with other values such as loyalty to friends, need for employment, political sensitivity, professional aspirations, and public relations impact' (King and Baxter Magolda, 1996, p. 167).

Ethical reasoning involves such moral character as ego strength, perseverance, resoluteness, strength of convictions, ability to resist distractions and overcome frustrations, and the ability to carry through on a moral course of action (Rest and Narvaez, 1994). All of these attributes are called upon in decision making in the 'messy swamp' of health care's ill-defined problems, which must be waded through for the benefit of the patient in a particular situation. Ethical reasoning includes pragmatic considerations in treatment, client-centred reasoning, and the therapist's beliefs and personal schema.

Pragmatic considerations in treatment

Neuhaus (1988) reports that therapists are often challenged to consider the ethical dilemmas or implications of their work when they are required to incorporate pragmatic influences into treatment planning. Therapists use this type of reasoning to decide what can be done for a particular patient in a given treatment setting (Schell and Cervero, 1993). With pragmatic reasoning, therapists consider the impact of personal and practice constraints on clinical decision making in everyday situations (Mattingly and Fleming, 1994; Schell and Cervero, 1993). It includes the therapist's personal paradigm (internal personal factors), all the practical issues that affect occupational therapy services, the treatment environment, the therapist's values, knowledge, abilities and experiences, the patient's social and financial resources, and the patient's potential discharge environment.

Client-centred reasoning

Ethical principles include respect for the individual and imply that any treatment provided should not interfere with the patient's personal and cultural values. In occupational therapy, the patient is the change agent and this person's active participation is required in determining and prioritising goals, thus gaining a sense of self-determination, control and commitment to treatment goals. Ethical treatment requires value judgement and the ability to empower the patient by providing options, explaining outcomes and outlining a time sequence. The rights of the family and the values and resources available may limit the choices the patient and therapist can make (Rogers, 1983).

Therapist's beliefs and personal schema

Health care practitioners may be influenced by their own emotional or subjective response to a particular circumstance, suggesting that they are not 'value-free' and they may have biases related to age, gender, race, religion, or even some past experience with particular patients (Woolley, 1990). These responses may dramatically affect the standard of care of the patient and create ethical concerns for the patient, the professional and the clinical setting. Therapists may inadvertently use themselves as the model for the view of the patient, ascribing meaning to the patient's situation from the perspective of the therapist's own reality. Clinical reasoning may thus be misdirected. Context affects our ability to implement knowledge based on information and affects our choice of tasks and tools (White and Stancombe, 2003).

Challenges to clinical reasoning raised by complex patient cases are common. Time pressures, reduced patient length of stay, workload demands and expectations of employers all impact on the quality of clinical reasoning. Benamy (1996) identifies a number of causes of common errors in clinical reasoning performed inadvertently by therapists. These include early hypothesis generation, expectations and inaccurate assumptions made by the therapist regarding their patient and an over-reliance on standard techniques. The value of peer review and supervision is a common way for therapists to review these challenges and devise effective strategies.

These aspects of reasoning are an attempt to explain the wide perspective of interaction between the therapist and the patient and the ongoing process of the therapy situation. It incorporates the use of knowledge, the action of cognition or thinking, and the process of meta-cognition. This process becomes more proficient as the therapist gains clinical experience. Research shows that occupational therapists, however, are not always aware of the use of clinical reasoning strategies. How therapists reason is reported to be influenced by their area of practice, their clinical experience and the stage at which they are treating the patient (Chapparo and Ranka, 2000).

Results of analysis based on matrix

The development of levels extends from the novices' reasoning based on a lack of ability to respond adequately to information presented (Roberts, 1996), and extends on to the expert therapist's ability to use intuitive thinking to develop goals based on patients' needs. Therapists in this study were found to range over the spectrum from advanced beginner to expert. It was not expected that any would be at novice level as they had all worked more than two years in a clinical setting.

It was found that the expert therapists were more attuned to their clients, referred to their client's perspective more often and commented on their own clinical reasoning with reference to their clients rather than in general terms.

The therapists in this study demonstrated a good to excellent knowledge base in practical skill application but showed more difficulty in the interpersonal communication and client centredness overall. The data indicated that the higher level of reasoning, the clearer the interaction and explanation of interaction with the client.

In relation to the novice to expert scale, it was found, however, that therapists did not always fit into only one level of reasoning.

For example, one therapist might have a great deal of experience working in the field of pressure therapy and be considered proficient-to-expert in evidence discovery and theory application, but have the personal empathy and client-centred approach that might signify a lower level of ethical reasoning. This may indicate excellent professional knowledge of burns including the related body systems, healing mechanisms, and understanding of the physics of pressure to reduce hypertrophic scarring. It may signify the professional judgement to understand when more or less pressure is required. It might not, however, include the interpersonal skills, ability to explain and educate, understanding of psychological and emotional issues surrounding disfigurement and scarring, and all the skills that are necessary in any therapy situation which would signify a truly proficient or expert therapist. A therapist from this study who was providing pressure therapy for a young child with severe burns, was quick and intuitive in her cognitive thinking and theory application about the physical aspects of treatment of burns, but was not so expert in the personal interaction and responses to the child's mother.

In relation to the reflective judgement perspective of clinical reasoning, most of the therapists in this study were quasi-reflective in that they could accept ambiguity to a degree but were often protocol-led. They did not demonstrate the ability to justify treatment based on criteria such as weight of evidence, utility of solution, pragmatic need for action. They did not appear to be reflective on their practice and, in some cases, found the interview a new experience in reflection. Reflective judgement was incorporated into the matrix as a necessary component of clinical reasoning as it indicates the personal ability to weigh arguments and make 'best' decisions. Epistemological beliefs lay the foundation for judgement in all situations, including clinical encounters. Understanding one's own beliefs and biases is fundamental to developing into an expert reflective practitioner.

Novice students and therapists are dependent on theory and rules to guide thinking and actions, and can describe only textbook examples or known solutions to problems. They have however some life experience which will inform their understanding. For instance, any student or beginning therapist can identify a state of high agitation in a client without having to objectively measure change in heart rate. However, recognising multiples or varying causes, or assessing and treating a person to reduce this high agitation, requires more than just this basic awareness. Recognising a person's agitation is only the first step in understanding the person's problem in context and starting to deal with it by identifying relevant sources for information.

Advanced beginners are more aware of the situational nature of tasks and experiences and begin to recognise the complexity of a problem or task. This raised awareness includes an increased number of relevant elements and more complicated rules. As more competence and confidence is gained in practice, therapists gain more flexibility and creativity in understanding a client's circumstances and in prioritising issues. They become more adept at predicting multiple outcomes and coping with changing conditions.

Expert practitioners incorporate technical and procedural efficiency and effectiveness with values and ethics. Being flexible, organised, broadminded, honest and conscientious are some attributes suggested for the expert practitioner, which parallel that of the ideal critical thinker (Scheffer and Rubenfeld, 2000). Therapists' professional thinking and clinical reasoning involve judgement which incorporates an understanding of a person's experience with, and response to, an illness or disabling situation while at the same time understanding family concerns. Expert therapists attend to salient information, prioritise issues, are attuned to subtle changes in a clinical situation and make conscious deliberate decisions. Expert practitioners use 'knowing how' (skill component) and 'knowing that' (knowledge of procedures), knowing-in-action (Schön, 1983), and knowing the particular client in order to recognise and respond to particular circumstances. People's expertise is usually related to experience in an area or certain type of situation, e.g. working with dying patients, and understanding of technical or computer access for specific groups of clients. This expertise tends to be domain specific.

The decisions made by therapists are not straightforward, and cannot be easily described or delineated. They involve choice, deliberation and practicality. They may include decisions 'not' to act, decisions that are important but are often forgotten about. Decisions may involve 'reflection on' and 'reflection in' practice (Schön, 1983). Therapists must generate and weigh up alternative solutions and the consequences of those solutions if they are to be effective in practice. Integral to decision making and good judgement are the practical wisdom, the prudence (moral judgement) and the morally appropriate actions for every situation (Fish and Coles, 1998). These attributes could be applied to health care professionals at the high end of the matrix.

Summary and conclusion

The clinical reasoning process has been described as a largely tacit, highly imaginistic and deeply phenomenological mode of thinking aimed at determining the best for each particular patient (Chapparo and Ranka, 2000). It is based in the beliefs, attitudes and expectations held by the therapist. For occupational therapists, there is also a focus on the examination of the personal meaning of illness, disability and therapy action (Mattingly and Fleming, 1994). The expert practitioner incorporates all these facets in the understanding of the patient and the development and implementation of treatment.

Multiple reasoning strategies come into play in the various phases of patient treatment. Procedural reasoning is used when therapists think about the patient's problems in terms of disease and human occupation. Narrative reasoning involves developing an understanding of the patient as a person from the patient's perspective. Conditional reasoning allows the therapist to visualise the future and consider therapy outcomes and the treatment required to get there. Ethical and pragmatic reasoning frame decision making in the personal and professional context.

In practice, an occupational therapist could be using all of these reasoning strategies simultaneously when thinking about a patient and treatment, or may focus on one or more strategies at a particular moment during or after therapy. This implies that knowledge includes skills as well as procedures. The procedures are the guidelines for action, the 'know that', and the skills are the 'know how' as suggested by Dreyfus and Dreyfus (1986). The know-how mediates motor actions and is the by-product of knowledge in action and requires direct cognitive input (Bridge and Twible, 1997). Jones (1997) notes that the client's values and beliefs, individual physical, psychological, social and cultural presentation, and the environmental resources such as time, funding, or externally imposed requirements, affect how the therapist will make decisions. All these influences may be considered a source of knowledge, a deterrent or a motivation for decision making (Chapparo and Ranka, 2000).

This chapter describes the clinical reasoning undertaken by occupational therapists as identified in the research. The facets of clinical reasoning found to be part of the process were noted. Findings were integrated with other clinical reasoning research in occupational therapy and related health care fields. It is to be noted that the matrix is a simplification of the complex and often demanding issues that are considered within a complex and messy practical setting. These situations require decision making and judgement that can be routine simple choice based on the therapist's preference and shaped by the therapist's own visions and understanding. They may require rapid reactions that allow no time to reflect and may afterwards generate questions of how and why such decisions were made. They may be decisions that require long deliberation and best choice in a situation that has no best solution.

The final results of the analysis of therapists' data verified the facets of the matrix that were identified, and the stage development of the facets in the Sinclair Matrix of Clinical Reasoning. The matrix is a step-wise progression of the facets of clinical reasoning for occupational therapy practice through the stages of development towards competence and expertise. It provides a framework for reflecting on the requirements for clinical reasoning in best practice. It demonstrates levels of development of facets of clinical reasoning based on the combination of personal values, professional knowledge and skills, cognitive skills, with life and clinical experience. It can be used in the assessment of competence and as a holistic framework for professional development. Using the Sinclair Matrix of Clinical Reasoning can act as a powerful tool in education and in practice.

References

Alnervik, A. and Sviden, G. (1996) On clinical reasoning: patterns of reflection on practice. *Occupational Therapy Journal of Research*, **16**(2), 98–110.

Argyris, C. and Schon, D. (1974) *Theory in Practice: Increasing Professional Effectiveness*, Jossey-Bass, San Francisco.

Benamy, B.C. (1996) *Developing Clinical Reasoning Skills: Strategies for the Occupational Therapist*, Therapy Skill Builders, San Antonio, TX.

Benner, P. (1984) *From Novice to Expert: Excellence and Power in Clinical Nursing Practice*, Addision-Wesley, Menlo Park, CA.

Boshuizen, H.P.A. and Schmidt, H.G. (1995) The development of clinical reasoning expertise, in *Clinical Reasoning in Health Science* (eds J. Higgs and M. Jones), Butterworth-Heinemann Ltd, Oxford, pp. 15–22.

Bridge, C. and Twible, R. (1997) Clinical reasoning: informed decision making for practice, in *Occupational Therapy: Enabling Function and Well-being* (eds C. Christiansen and C. Baum), Slack, Thorofare, NJ, pp. 160–79.

Carr, W. (1995) *For Education: Towards Critical Educational Enquiry*, Open University Press, London.

Chapparo, C. and Ranka, J. (2000) Clinical reasoning in occupational therapy, in *Clinical Reasoning in the Health Professions* (eds J. Higgs and M. Jones), Butterworth-Heinemann Ltd, Oxford, pp. 128–37.

Crabtree, M. (1998) Images of reasoning: a literature review. *Australian Occupational Therapy Journal*, **45**, 113–23.

Dreyfus, H.L. and Dreyfus, S.E. (1986) *Mind over Machine*, Collier Macmillan, Inc., New York.

Dutton, R. (1995) *Clinical Reasoning in Physical Disabilities*, Williams & Wilkins, Baltimore, MD.

Fish, D. and Coles, C. (1998) *Developing Professional Judgement in Health Care*, Butterworth-Heinemann, Oxford.

Fleming, M.H. (1991) The therapist with the three-track mind. *American Journal of Occuapational Therapy*, **45**(11), 1007–14.

Fortmeier, S. and Thanning, G. (2002) *From the Patient's Point of View*, Ergoterapeutforeningen, Copenhagen.

Higgs, J., Richardson, B. and Dahlgren, M.A. (2004) *Developing Practice Knowledge for Health Professionals*, Butterworth Heinemann, Edinburgh.

Hooper, B. (1997) The relationship between pretheoretical assumptions and clinical reasoning. *American Journal of Occupational Therapists*, **51**(5), 328–38.

Jones, M. (1997) Clinical reasoning: the foundation of clinical practice. Part 1. *Australian Journal of Physiotherapy*, **43**(3), 167–70.

King, P.M. and Baxter Magolda, M.B. (1996) A developmental perspective on learning. *Journal of College Student Development*, **37**(2), 163–73.

King, P.M. and Kitchner, K.S. (1985) Reflective judgement theory and research: insights into the process of knowing in the college gess. Paper presented at the Annual Meeting of the American College Personnel Association, Boston.

Mattingly, C. (1991) The narrative nature of clinical reasoning. *American Journal of Occupational Therapy*, **45**, 998–1005.

Mattingly, C. and Fleming, M.H. (1994) *Clinical Reasoning: Forms of Inquiry in a Therapeutic Practice*, F.A. Davis Co., Philadelphia.

Neistadt, M.E., Wight, J. and Mulligan, S.E. (1998) Clinical reasoning case studies as teaching tools. *American Journal of Occupational Therapy*, **52**(2), 125–32.

Neuhaus, B.E. (1988) Ethical considerations in clinical reasoning: the impact of technology and cost containment. *American Journal of Occupational Therapy*, **42**(5), 288–94.

Perkins, D.N. (1987) Thinking frames: an integrative perspective on teaching cognitive skills. *Teaching Thinking Skills: Theory and Practice* (eds J.B. Baron and R.J. Sternberg), Freeman, New York, pp. 41–61.

Reed, K. and Sanderson, S. (1999) *Concepts of Occupational Therapy*, Lippincott, Williams & Wilkins, Baltimore, MD.

Rest, J.R. and Narvaez, D. (1994) *Moral Development in the Professions: Psychology and Applied Ethics*, Lawrence Erlbaum Associates, Hillsdale, NJ.

Roberts, A.E. (1996) Clinical reasoning in occupational therapy: idiosyncrasies in content and process. *British Journal of Occupational Therapy*, **59**(8), 372–6.

Rogers, J.C. (1983) Clinical reasoning: the ethics, science and art. *American Journal of Occupational Therapy*, **37**, 601–16.

Rogers, J.C. (1986) Clinical judgment: the bridge between theory and practice, in *Target 2000: Occupational Therapy Education*, American Occupational Therapy Association, Rockville, MD.

Scheffer, B.K. and Rubenfeld, M.G. (2000) A consensus statement on critical thinking in nursing. *Journal of Nursing Education*, **39**(8), 352–9.

Schell, B.A. and Cervero, R.M. (1993) Clinical reasoning in occupational therapy: an integrative review. *American Journal of Occupational Therapy*, **47**(7), 605–10.

Schon, D. (1983) *The Reflective Practitioner: How Professionals Think in Action*, Basic Books, New York.

Schwartzberg, S.L. (2002) *Interative Reasoning in the Practice of Occupational Therapy*, Pearson Education, Upper Saddle River, NJ.

Smith, R. (1992) Theory: an entitlement to understanding. *Cambridge Journal of Education*, **22**: 387–98.

White, S. and Stancombe, J. (2003) *Clinical Judgement in the Health and Welfare Professions*, Open University Press, Maidenhead, UK.

Woolley, N. (1990) Nursing diagnosis: exploring the factors which may influence the reasoning process. *Journal of Advanced Nursing*, **15**, 110–17.

Knowing more than we can say

9

Priscilla Harries

Introduction

For the past ten years I have been researching how occupational therapists make wise clinical judgements. The reasons for this are threefold: by making our thinking explicit we can study our decisions, we can identify good judgements and we can shape our professional theories. Values that influence our reasoning can be shared and developed. The knowledge gained from researching our clinical reasoning also has important implications for occupational therapy education and practice.

The specific area I focus on relates to how occupational therapists make judgements of referral priorities in community mental health teams. I was initially interested in how referral information is used and how it influences the service provision. As my research progressed, issues of expertise and training entered the equation.

Community mental health is a particularly challenging field as there are many influential factors which impact on occupational therapists' judgements: extended scope practice, caseload management and the tension between generic working and occupationally focused working. Community service users are now more severely ill than two decades ago as there is less in-patient provision. This places a heavier demand on service providers and, if the skills of the workforce are not well matched to service demands, burnout can occur. Service providers have to provide an effective service that matches organisational, professional and personal values. These are not necessarily congruent, and professional values can be at odds with governmental policy. There may be only one occupational therapist in the mental health team, so she may lack guidance on how to successfully negotiate a path through these complex issues. We need to retain our workforce to have any chance of meeting the high level of need in the community. We need to know how experienced therapists make their judgements; how they identify and combine the information needed to make their judgements. This information can then be used to train novices.

My research led me to ask many questions: how do we make wise clinical judgements, how much insight do we have into our judgements, how capable are we of reflection, which policies should we be teaching novices and how can we teach expert thinking? In this chapter I will attempt to answer some of these questions using examples from the many occupational therapists who gave their time to share their clinical judgements.

The first part of the chapter will explain the issue of referral prioritisation and the rationale for studying this particular judgement process. I then present the judgement analysis study which I undertook to identify the prioritisation policies of 40 occupational therapists. The next part will give a critique of the early clinical reasoning studies, which mainly used information-processing methodologies. Two alternative methodologies will then be presented: the decision analysis approach and judgement analysis. The last part of the chapter will deal with issues of expertise development and self-insight; each topic being linked to my research endeavours into these topics.

The need for skills in referral prioritisation

In Britain, all health services are in short supply (Spalding, 1999). Priority setting is unfortunately necessary where demand for services exceeds service availability. In the field of mental health, the need to recruit and retain occupational therapists is high on occupational therapy managers' agendas (Craik *et al.*, 1999). The need to maximise the effectiveness of services and minimise attrition of occupational therapists has become an international aim (Bailey, 1990; Sturgess and Poulsen, 1983). In community teams, occupational therapists can often be professionally isolated and some report that the needs of severely ill clients can take their toll on the therapist (Bassett and Lloyd, 2001). However, others report that they are providing an effective service and are satisfied that they have a valued role (Parker, 2001). It is apparent that research is needed to identify and share these methods of effective practice.

One issue of effective practice for community mental health practitioners is the ability to balance responsibilities for professionally skilled intervention with generic care co-ordination responsibilities. Where generic responsibilities are time consuming, there can be little time given to professionally skilled interventions. The combination of providing care co-ordination alongside specialist services concerns the occupational therapy profession (Corrigan, 2002; Forsyth and Summerfield Mann, 2002; Harries, 2002). In Britain, the College of Occupational Therapists has identified that occupational therapists need to focus the majority of their time on clients requiring occupational therapy (Craik *et al.*, 1998a). Therefore, when taking responsibility for care co-ordination, occupational therapists have to consider whether clients would best benefit from an occupational therapy perspective. Those referrals that require occupational therapy intervention must then be prioritised according to degree of occupational dysfunction. These dysfunctions may be in the occupational areas of self-care, work/productivity or leisure (Reed and Sanderson, 1992). Skill in prioritising referrals in this way maximises the effectiveness of services at a time of staff shortages.

In order to prioritise effectively, occupational therapists have to develop appropriate prioritisation policies both for prioritising direct occupational therapy referrals and for team referrals. Once they accept a client onto their caseload they have responsibility for that client and they may not be able to have the case reallocated. If they accept inappropriate referrals, they may be unable to manage their clients' needs effectively or they may feel their skills are not being used satisfactorily. The stress of this situation can lead to burnout (Craik *et al.*, 1998b). To avoid this, therapists need to have specific expertise and feel confident that they are making a useful contribution. Taking appropriate referrals therefore has two potential benefits: it ensures effective use of professional services and also improves work satisfaction.

Judgements are one component of clinical reasoning; they influence what type of information is counted as important (and therefore paid attention to) and how much weight that information needs to be given. When prioritisation decisions are made, judgements have to be used to recognise what information leads to higher or lower levels of prioritisation. Research into occupational therapists' ability to examine referral data is not new (Grime, 1990; Harries, 1996a, 1998; Job 1996). However, formal research on clinical reasoning in occupational therapy has mainly been qualitative in nature, often using the information-processing approach (Newell and Simon, 1972). In addition, only small samples of clinicians' prioritisation policies have been accessed, thus reducing possibilities for generalisability (Hagedorn, 1996; Harries, 1996a, b; Munroe, 1996; Roberts, 1996). If research were done on a larger scale, experts' policies could be used as evidence for clinical education, ensuring that new knowledge would be up to date and, hence, effective in meeting clients' needs (Lloyd-Smith, 1997). Good practice could then be shared in order to promote effective services for the client (Department of Health, 1999). When considering what methodology would be appropriate to investigate clinical reasoning, the literature was key. Much of this had been influenced by American clinical studies that had used mainly qualitative methodologies (Elstein *et al.*, 1978; Fleming, 1991a, b; Mattingly, 1991). This chapter will return to the issue of research methodologies at a later stage.

The next section describes the study of the referral prioritisation policies of experienced therapists and the nature of those policies. These policies are then discussed in relation to the types of work practices the therapists were undertaking. Issues of specific roles and generic working are key to this. To see the full method and results of this study, the reader is referred to Harries and Gilhooly (2003a).

Occupational therapists' referral prioritisation policies

In 2000–01, 40 occupational therapists with experience of working in the field of community mental health were asked to make decisions on the priority of 90 referrals. Thirty repeat referrals were added to the set to check for test-retest reliability. An example of a referral is shown in Figure 9.1. Factors which had the potential to influence the degree of priority given were randomised into the computer-generated referrals, using Visual Basic as the programming tool. Therapists could potentially use nine types of information on the form as a cue to the level of priority of the referral, for example, the client's diagnosis. At the foot of the referral form a horizontal line (visual analogue scale) labelled low priority at one end and high priority at the other end enabled participants to indicate their rating of the priority of the referral by making a cross somewhere along the line. Individual participants' ratings were collected for each referral presented and the mean group rating for each referral was calculated across participants by adding the ratings for each profile and dividing by 40.

The results showed that the most important cue, used by three-quarters of the occupational therapists, was the reason for referral. This was encouraging, as this is usually where cue information about the degree of occupational dysfunction is described. The second most used cue was history of violence and the third was diagnosis. In this research, history of violence included suicide risk. Suicide prevention is part of a larger governmental prioritisation policy (Department of Health, 1995) and community mental health teams, who have an important role in helping to reduce the suicide rate, are encouraged to support this policy. Diagnosis also gives indirect information as to the nature of the occupational dysfunction. For example, schizophrenia is recognised as having a more detrimental effect on occupational functioning than other diagnoses such as anxiety and depression. Clients with schizophrenia often have difficulties around self-care, concentration, motivation, use of time, occupational balance and socialisation. These difficulties commonly benefit from an occupational perspective

Community Occupational Therapy Mental Health Referral Form (Adult Mental Health Services)

Client's name	*Mr xx*	Address *Within catchment area.*
Age	*48* D.o.b *xx/xx/xx*	
Date of referral	*xx/xx/xx (Recent)*	
Name of referrer	*GP*	Telephone *(xxxx) xxx xxxx*
Consultant	*Dr xx*	GP *Dr xx*

Diagnosis *Anxiety* *Five year history*

Current living situation

Home with family

Reason for referral

Psychological and physical disabilities. Functional assessment needed to identify level of support required.

Other services involved

Counsellor

Any known history of violence? *Physically abusive*

Is the client aware of the referral? *Yes*

Low priority   High priority

Figure 9.1   Example of referral

(Creek, 1990), therefore schizophrenia draws the particular attention of the occupational therapist.

A cluster analysis was then conducted to compare therapists' policies. Four subgroups of occupational therapists were identified, each using a different type of policy from the other three subgroups. The methodology also allowed for consistency in prioritisation to be measured, as repeated referrals were included among the set. One subgroup had a very low consistency score, that is, they marked identical referrals as low and high priority within the one-hour task. Demographic and practice data were also collected on all participants. These data were used to see if there was any type of policy linked to a particular type of individual or practice setting. The four groups were found to differ from each other according to five factors: the percentage of role dedicated to specialist occupational therapy or generic work, satisfaction with the balance in these roles, the number of hours worked, the number of professionally trained team members and the presence of referral prioritisation policies.

Using demographic data to differentiate the groups, a name was allocated to each one: the aspiring specialists, the satisfied specialists, the satisfied genericists and the chameleons. The aspiring specialists were unhappy with the large amount of generic working they were expected to do and the majority of their caseload was linked to generic working. The satisfied specialists were fairly happy with their caseload balance and they spent the majority of their time on occupational-therapy-specific work. The satisfied genericists spend the majority of their time on generic casework and were satisfied with the caseload balance. The chameleons were those who had the lowest scores in consistent application of policy because they did not apply a specific policy consistently.

From the demographic data, one of the most important findings was that half of the occupational therapists felt their caseload was too large, yet they were accepting the majority of their direct referrals as well as a proportion of team referrals. Half of the occupational therapists felt that they had too much responsibility for generic casework. On average, they had care co-ordination responsibilities for 64% of the clients on their caseload. All but one occupational therapist had a care co-ordinator role, but only one-third of therapists in this role were taking occupational therapy specific referrals only.

The satisfied generalists and the satisfied specialists were fairly satisfied with their caseload balance and both subgroups were providing a service that they saw as highly valued. Perhaps the group of occupational therapists who are most at risk of leaving their posts and, potentially, the profession, which was the largest subgroup, are the aspiring specialists who felt least satisfied with their caseload balance. This group do not use the policies that orientate their casework to working with clients with occupational need (Craik *et al.*, 1998b).

Care co-ordination has benefits for clients, such as ensuring that responsibility is taken by one individual for the comprehensive assessment and provision of services to a client. Occupational therapists support this client-centred approach as opposed to one that is professionally centred (Corrigan, 2002). However, due to the relatively small number of occupational therapists in community mental health teams, occupational therapists may be in a difficult position if they give the majority of their time to generic casework. It appears that the role the profession advocates, that of having a majority of casework focusing on occupational need, may be the optimal balance for occupational therapists to take. Perhaps in this way occupational therapists' skills can be best used and clients' needs most effectively met.

It was clear that the type of policy that led to the occupational therapist taking more of a specialist role gave particular importance to the reason for referral and the client's diagnosis. Policies that led to mainly generic working gave greatest importance to potential violence or suicide risk. When talking to therapists at the conference of the Association of Occupational Therapists in Mental Health, in

April 2003, support was found for this rationale. Those who wished to work generically sought out referrals that would require a high level of crisis intervention support. Occupational therapists who wished to maintain more of an occupational therapy service actively avoided crisis intervention referrals.

Many occupational therapists would agree that they can assist clients to find meaning in their life and, hence, reduce the wish to commit suicide, but is it perhaps the role of other team members to reduce suicide risk when working in the community? If clients are at risk to themselves or others they may need to be sectioned under the Mental Health Act 1983 (Department of Health, 1983). In this case, the community psychiatric nurse, psychiatrist or social worker has the authority to hospitalise clients and may therefore be best suited to managing suicidal crises. If clients have the acute symptoms of psychosis or depression, they may need medication, and knowledge of medication benefits is more within the field of expertise of the community psychiatric nurse or the psychiatrist rather than the occupational therapist.

The participants in this study were sampled from all over the UK and were all working in separate teams. It was, therefore, not surprising that the types of cue they used to make their prioritisation decisions varied widely. Some placed most emphasis on the reason for referral whereas others used history of violence as the most important cue. However, when examining how they used the content of the cues, such as the different types of diagnosis, there was very good agreement on what influenced prioritisation. For example, 88% gave people with a diagnosis of schizophrenia the highest priority. A total of 93% gave a high priority to those people living alone as opposed to those living with family or in group homes. All therapists gave the highest priority to those people with no support as opposed to those seeing a counsellor or having a day centre place. A total of 83% used suicidal behaviour as a higher priority for service than physical or verbal aggression to others. These results indicate that the *National Service Framework for Mental Health* priorities (Department of Health, 1999) for serious illness and suicidal intentions are being consistently used and prioritised by occupational therapists. Only two therapists used length of history of illness in their prioritisation policies, giving priority to those people with shorter histories rather than longer histories and appearing not to take account of the *National Service Framework* priorities that relate to long-term mental health problems. Perhaps taking some clients with shorter histories is preferred if there is perceived to be a greater potential for positive change. If the therapist has a caseload of long-term severely ill clients, some clients with shorter histories may be considered better prospects for intervention (Bassett and Lloyd, 2001).

The primary purpose of this research was to elicit how experienced occupational therapists prioritise their services. However, the sampling criteria did not guarantee that participants were experts in clinical reasoning. Their length of time working as a community occupational therapist, membership of a special interest group and seniority of grade did not ensure that they had policies that were consistently applied. For example, when one participant's ratings on the original and repeat referrals were correlated, she was found to have poor consistency in applying her prioritisation policy ($r = 0.29$). When a policy is inconsistently applied, this is a sign of limited expertise (Shanteau, 2001).

Clinical reasoning research: the start

In terms of medical research, Arthur Elstein and his colleagues conducted the first major studies into clinical decision making (Elstein *et al.*, 1978). The original studies used three methods of data collection: direct observation of problem solving using simulated clinical problems, concurrent think aloud and retrospection (while viewing video footage) (Elstein *et al.*, 1978). The aims of the study were three-fold: to identify experts' reasoning processes, to consider the context of these theories in relation to individuals' attributes and existing psychological theories and to develop direction for future medical education. The findings identified a type of reasoning, described as hypothetico-deductive reasoning, which was found to involve a process of generating and testing hypotheses.

The first major study to explore the reasoning strategies of occupational therapists was published in 1991. This study was sponsored by the American Occupational Therapy Association (AOTA) and the American Occupational Therapy Foundation (AOTF) (Fleming, 1991a, b; Mattingly, 1991). It used an ethnographic and action research approach in which seventeen occupational therapists were interviewed, observed and videoed over a two-year period. The researchers identified reasoning tracks or styles and linked these to reasoning strategies. They incorporated the work of Donald Schön (1983) who placed value on reflection as a means of understanding implicit or tacit reasoning (Mattingly and Fleming, 1994).

The researchers in the AOTA/AOTF study argued that the specific style of occupational therapists' reasoning is dependent on the content of the task being thought about (Mattingly and Fleming, 1994). For example, if a clinician is thinking about occupational dysfunction, a style named procedural reasoning is used (Fleming, 1991b). Thought relating to a client's perspective of their needs was termed interactive reasoning and thought relating to a client's context and future potential was termed conditional reasoning (Fleming, 1991b). The findings also identified other reasoning strategies such as 'narrative reasoning' (Mattingly, 1991). The findings of this study appear to have greatly influenced later clinical reasoning studies in the field of occupational therapy. Subsequent research on tracks of reasoning in occupational therapy sometimes classified verbalised thoughts by type of task content (Fortune and Ryan, 1996; Fossie, 1996). At times this could appear a little forced. For example, questions relating to future prognosis were purposely asked to elicit conditional reasoning (Alvervik and Sviden, 1996; Ryan, 1990).

The AOTA/AOTF study also searched for evidence of reasoning processes previously identified in the fields of psychology and medicine. Hypothetico-deductive strategies (Schmidt et al., 1990) were thought to be used primarily in procedural reasoning and intuitive strategies were thought to be used primarily in interactive reasoning (Fleming, 1991b). Mattingly and Fleming may not have meant their findings, linking thought content with thinking process, to be understood in such a purist light. Indeed, in their book published in 1994 they were able to give greater depth to the understanding of the nature of the reasoning strategies used. However, the content/process link seems to have been grasped firmly and applied to much of the recent occupational therapy research. As a result of this, many researchers have classified occupational therapists' clinical reasoning either by the thought content (e.g. procedural) or by the reasoning strategies recognised in the thought processing (e.g. hypothetico-deductive) (Alvervik and Sviden, 1996).

Identifying experts' clinical judgements

In 1995, qualitative data on the reasoning of community mental health occupational therapists was collected in order to examine the factors influencing their acceptance of referrals (Harries, 1996a). Following the lead of Mattingly and Fleming, methodologies drawn from the qualitative paradigm were used, more specifically those within the information-processing approach. Clinicians were asked to think aloud as they read real referral letters. This verbalisation was then transcribed and analysed for themes or thinking strategies. Although this method could potentially increase the time of the thinking task, the method itself was known not to lead to any changes in the actual judgements or decisions (Ericsson and Simon, 1980). These think alouds were then followed immediately with individual in-depth interviews.

The findings, drawn from vocalised think-aloud data, showed several points of interest. Participants had their own personal methods of framing the data. This was seen through the way in which they always attended to two or three particular factors, regardless of the referral information.

Although the think-aloud method accessed some points of interest, the process-tracing methodology also had weaknesses. Firstly, the think aloud did not access all the thinking that had occurred. For example, the participant would read the client's diagnosis but make no further comment. However, in the subsequent interview there was lengthy explanation about the relevance of the client's diagnosis. This disparity may be explained by the recognition that the experienced clinician uses minimal processing to make sense of familiar information (Abernathy and Hamm, 1994).

Another weakness of the think-aloud method related to the difficulty in understanding which vocalised thoughts were relevant to the decision task under study and which were not. For example, it was only through the interview that it became apparent that some thoughts related to the decision to accept or reject the case while others related to issues such as treatment planning. It is not surprising that the decision to accept the case was intertwined with other thinking tasks: other researchers have found that experienced clinicians do not use each stage of the occupational therapy process in a linear pattern (one stage following another) but rather in a much more complex way (Hagedorn, 1996; Roberts, 1996). Had the think aloud been used without the interview, the purpose of the reasoning would not have become apparent.

However, the most concerning issue was that factors mentioned in the think alouds were not always acknowledged in the interviews. For example, when occupational therapists were asked how they took account of their referral sources, such as the family doctor or psychiatrist, they stated that the referral source was not important, as the referral priority would depend on the client's type of occupational dysfunction. However, some participants, when asked to do a concurrent think aloud on three new referrals, clearly took account of the referral source and let it influence their decision as to whether or not to accept a referral. For example, some subjects felt they had to accept the referral when the referrer was in a position of power:

> umm. Usually if my consultant writes me a letter I have to take it anyway but still . . .
>
> (Harries, 1996a, p. 57)

If they had a good relationship with the referrer they would also be encouraged to accept the referral:

> but I would probably [accept this] if this was one of our CPNs [community psychiatric nurses]. I would take this on face value as we have a good relationship between us in terms of clients that we see and I would arrange to go and visit this guy purely based on the fact that my colleague suggested that he thinks I might be able to help this person.
>
> (Harries, 1996a, p. 57)

The qualitative interview method therefore appeared to encourage reflection on tacit knowledge. This type of knowledge is not readily accessible to the participant and can be difficult to describe accurately. This appeared to lead to some disparity between individuals' actual practice policies and their reported policies. At this point the literature was used again to look for explanations and to search for other methodologies that could lead to better understanding of how the thinking of experienced therapists could be elicited. Elstein's ten-year retrospective of their results from their medical studies was found to be relevant (Elstein *et al.*, 1990). They too had found conflicting information from their three data sources. They decided that data should be weighted in the following order: direct observation of problem solving using simulated clinical problems, concurrent think aloud and retrospection (Elstein *et al.*, 1990). Concurrent think alouds were given more weight than retrospection. Although this suggestion may have been based on some post-hoc rationalisation, the think alouds were therefore considered to have more validity than interviews. They were concurrent rather than retrospective, which helped to reduce issues such as accuracy of recall. It was noted that the proponents of another school of thought, the decision analysis theorists, were also interested in the individual's lack of ability to explain accurately their own policies. Their perspective was examined to establish whether their methods were going to be useful in making clinical decisions explicit.

The decision analysis approach

This approach came to the fore in 1954, when Paul Meehl published a review of 20 studies comparing intuitive clinical judgements and statistical combinations of the same information. His seminal book showed that, even on simple tasks, statistical methods were more accurate than human judgement (Meehl, 1954). A need to study clinical decisions through statistical means was advocated at the time and behavioural researchers took up this challenge aided, in the 1960s, by the arrival of computers (Elstein and Schwartz, 2000). This allowed tasks of human decision making and judgement to be statistically analysed and modelled to depths that had previously been limited (Arkes and Hammond, 1986). Decision analysis was now considered limitless. By the 1970s, decision-making research was increasing rapidly in the clinical field.

It is relevant to give some detail of the decision analysis approach at this point. Decision analysis is a quantitative approach to understanding decision making. It draws on theories from operation research, game theory, microeconomics and utility theory (Dawson and Cebul, 1990). The majority of medical decision analysis is based on expected utility theory (EUT) (Hershey and Baron, 1987). The likelihood of an event occurring is represented by a probability value and the desirability of the outcome is represented by a utility value. The component parts of the decision are then multiplied together to suggest a decision. All these factors are represented in a decision tree.

Where no objective probability values are available, an individual's beliefs of the probability of the expected outcome (subjective probabilities) can be used (subjectively expected model) (Savage, 1954). These two utility models, expected utility theory and subjective expected utility theory, were developed to describe decisions that contain an element of risk. Clinical decision making was categorised as risky, since the outcomes of clinical decisions are commonly unknown at the time the decision is made.

Decision analysis is viewed as a prescriptive or normative approach to understanding decisions, as it attempts to analyse the decision before it takes place and to suggest how decisions *should* be made. The type of information that decision analysis can yield was thought to have great potential for assisting clinicians. Probability statistics could be used to provide data for clinical guidelines, which would aid screening and treatment decisions (Hershey and Baron, 1987).

Cognitive theorists viewed decision analysis outcomes as superior to those of human cognition (Elstein, 1976). They felt that clinicians' decisions were unhelpfully influenced by cognitive bias (Dawson, 1987), which they viewed as detrimental to both human information synthesis and probability estimates (Dawson, 1993). They felt that clinical decisions should be based on quantitative knowledge of the effectiveness of treatment, chance of survival, cost effectiveness and the patient's resulting quality of life (Dawson and Cebul, 1990). They expected that clinicians and patients alike would recognise the superior value of formal decision analysis and would welcome the opportunity to use such valuable information, but this was not to be the case.

Cognitive theorists found clinicians very resistant to attempts to introduce decision aids (Elstein, 1976). Clinicians felt that the calculations of decision analysis were unmanageable and time consuming, and they had little faith in the validity of the analyses themselves. Clinicians were not sure that the probability figures had been derived from appropriate or accurate information and were also concerned that such quantitative approaches negated the intuitive nature of their decisions (Elstein, 1976).

Decision analysts attempted to remedy some of the clinicians' criticisms of their theories while continuing to promote the value of their work (Dawson, 1987). But, by the 1980s, the medical decision-making community still had little success in having its research incorporated into the daily lives of clinicians and it began to be less confident about the contribution it could make to clinical decision making. Community members felt outnumbered by clinicians and swamped by the vast number of medical decisions that needed to be understood before sufficient data could be provided (Fryback, 1983). At the same time, behavioural decision theorists had begun to show that the axioms of expected utility theory, although sounding plausible, actually differed from how clinicians reason (Tversky and Kahneman, 1981). This demonstrated that humans are not always rational and that utility probabilities will not necessarily lead clinicians to the decisions that the decision analysts would have expected. It was therefore acknowledged that expected utility theories were not going to be descriptive of how decisions were made in clinical practice (Hershey and Baron, 1987).

As probability-based decision support systems continued to remain unpopular with the majority of clinicians, knowledge-based information systems began to take their place. Knowledge-based systems were developed to provide rules or small units of information written in text. This form of information was more acceptable to clinicians. Instead of using probabilities, the system would ask the clinician questions and then use logic to draw a conclusion from the knowledge base (Fox and Alvey, 1983). It was thought that, at a minimal level, knowledge-based systems would be used to confirm clinicians' decisions (Fox and Alvey, 1983) but, as time is short in clinical settings, clinicians tend to rely on their own knowledge rather than checking with a computer database. Knowledge-based systems have also been used to provide the general public with a telephone advice service, NHS Direct (Department of Health, 2000). If systems are not used, it is unlikely that the information in them will be updated, due to the vast costs incurred (Gordon, 1991). The value of knowledge-based systems therefore appears limited in terms of the time it takes to develop them, the time it takes to use them and the cost of updating them. If this method is to be successful it will need to be accessible and easily understandable (Hoffrage *et al.*, 2000).

Decision analysts continued to hold differing views from information-processing theorists and criticised the methodology of process tracing. Although their own methods have flaws, they did not believe that process-tracing methodologies have the ability to describe the true decision-making process either. Their rationale for this criticism was that the importance of cues described in verbal protocols does not correlate, when compared with decision outcomes, to the weights given to those cues. Decision analysts felt that verbalisations were not a valid method of describing the full spectrum of thinking because they lacked the aspect of intuitive thought. This tension between normative and descriptive theorists was very apparent in the 1980s and 1990s, but neither camp appeared to have all the answers.

In 1993, a special issue of the journal *Cognition* was devoted to decision analysis, in an attempt to forge co-operation between the theorists. This went some way towards informing both camps about each other's fields. It did not appear that decision analysis was the methodology that would suit my own research.

I looked at a third group of theorists who had turned their attention to applying a different methodology: that of judgement analysis.

Judgement analysis

Judgement analysis usually involves studying individuals' decisions on a large number of scenarios in order to study how information has been used. By comparing the judgements made with the information (cues) that has been presented, a model of the decision-maker's judgements can be statistically produced. This model represents the decision-maker's tacit judgement policy. Judgement analysis has been used to study many fields, for example: how weather forecasters use their information to forecast imminent weather conditions (Stewart *et al.*, 1992) and how doctors use test results and clinical histories to judge whether to prescribe medication (Harries, 1995).

Judgement analysis was developed from three theories: probabilistic functionalism, social judgement theory and cognitive continuum theory (Cooksey, 1996).

Probabilistic functionalism was the idea of Egon Brunswik (1903–55), an Austrian-American psychologist (Doherty and Kurz, 1996). It was born from a concern that research into cognition was mainly experimental and that situations presented to subjects lacked the natural inter-cue correlations that would be found in the environment. Brunswik emphasised that situations must be based on the types of information that occur in the natural environment (Brunswik, 1952).

Brunswik felt that existing research had sampled subjects effectively but had neglected to sample the environment with the same care. The interaction between the individual and the environment, both in the individual's perception of the environment and in her or his response to that perception (functional response), is probabilistic (unpredictable) and therefore research needs to examine people's (or other organisms') perceptions in a wide range of possible situations.

A study by Tape *et al.* (1991) demonstrated the importance of the probabilistic structure of the environment. The researchers found that the accuracy of physicians' judgements about the probability of pneumonia in their patients, as measured through comparing X-ray results, was higher for physicians in Nebraska than in Virginia or Illinois. However, accuracy should be measured not only from the point of view of the decision maker but also in context of the predictability of the environment. When the environment was studied it was found that X-ray results had a clearer relationship to the symptoms in Nebraska than in Illinois and Virginia. Physicians' use of information in making their judgements was appropriate for the environment (the set of cases) in which they practised.

Brunswik's concern for ensuring that the environment was appropriately represented also extended to the subjects. Traditionally, experimental design aims to discover general laws by averaging results across subjects and finding trends in data. Instead, Brunswik advocated an idiographic-statistical approach (Brunswik, 1952) that requires analysis to be conducted on each individual in a range of situations. Brunswik's interest lay in finding, for each individual, the relationship between environmental cues and functional response. This relationship was viewed as the level of achievement or success in correctly using information to interpret what was actually occurring in the environment.

The second theory underpinning judgement analysis is social judgement theory. This was developed by Kenneth Hammond, a former student of Brunswik (Hammond *et al.*, 1975), who took Brunswik's ideas on perception in the physical environment and applied them to the study of human judgement within the social environment.

Hammond identified how correlation statistics (r being the correlation coefficient) could be used to determine how well a judge used the available information. In Hammond's adapted model, achievement or success in making an appropriate judgement (r_a) is the correlation between the individual's judgements (Y_s) with that which is being judged (Y_e). For example, how successfully a doctor accurately diagnosed (Y_s) the presenting symptoms (Y_e) can be represented by the statistic r_a. In correlation statistics, 1 indicates a perfect match (hence perfect success) and 0 means that there is no match (zero success). It is unlikely in risky decision-making situations, such as clinical decision making, that each extreme would occur but it is useful to identify where the judgement maker lies on the continuum in order to establish the accuracy of an individual's policy. How information is used by the individual and the accuracy of individuals' judgements are of great interest to judgement analysts.

They are also interested in the extent to which different individuals agree on the way information should be used. Therefore, following the identification of individual weighting policies (idiographic analysis), group-level analysis (nomothetic analysis) can be conducted to identify any groups of judges with similar policies. This is known as policy clustering (Cooksey, 1996).

The third theory underpinning the development of judgement analysis is cognitive continuum theory, which was also developed by Hammond (Cooksey, 1996). It focuses on a continuum between intuitive and analytical thinking. The five premises of cognitive continuum theory can be summarised as follows:

1. Forms of cognition are viewed along a continuum, the poles being represented by analytical thought and intuitive thought. The cognitive continuum index (CCI) is a method developed for quantifying the position of the decision maker along this continuum.

2. The mode of cognition between the poles is described as quasi-rational thought. This is composed of a mixture of both analytical and intuitive thought of differing proportions. No position on the continuum reflects a mode superior to any other point.

3. Characteristics of the judgement or decision tasks (complexity of task structure, ambiguity of task content, form of task presentation) induce the form of cognition. These characteristics also form another continuum, the task continuum index (TCI), which identifies the modes of thought that tasks are likely to induce. The TCI was developed to quantify the level of cognition likely to be induced by the different types of task.

4. The mode of cognition used by the decision maker is not static but can alter according to three influences: if a mode has been used successfully; if there has been previous experience of the task, or if the task characteristics change.

5. The CCI describes a range of cognitive modes from intuitive to analytic, with quasi-experimental processing as a midpoint. This continuum is in contrast to the dichotomy often drawn between processes that are implicit and unconscious and those that are explicit and fully conscious.

Analytical thinking is described as a slow, step-by-step, conscious, logical process in which cues are interpreted objectively and a formula is followed. Errors only occur if a mistake is made in the following steps. The individual's confidence in the method is therefore higher than in the outcome. Tasks that induce analytical thought include those where there are rules to follow, where the outcome is known and where there are less than five available cues.

Intuitive thinking is described as a fast, automated process in which the decision maker is not aware of how they arrive at the judgement. There is, therefore, low cognitive control (Hammond and Summers, 1972). As there is minimal conscious awareness of the thinking that has occurred, there can be little insight into that which has occurred. The individual's confidence is higher in the judgement than in the process. They may have a feeling that they have made a wise decision but cannot easily describe how they came to it.

Cognitive continuum theory does not assume, a priori, that either analysis or intuition is a superior mode of thought. In clinical judgements the mode of cognition is commonly a mixture of the two, analytical and intuitive (Hammond et al., 1975). However, when studying expert clinical judgement it is likely that the intuitive mode will be used, as past experience of the task is likely.

Studying how expert judgement has been made is not easy. It is important that the data collection method does not rely on the clinician's ability to make thinking strategies explicit. Judgement analysis has an advantage over process-tracing methods in that there is no requirement to access the processing stage; it is only required that clinicians make judgements or decisions as they normally would. The method does not rely on asking the decision maker to describe a decision-making process that may have become completely automatic and unconscious. Judgement analysis instead allows the use of statistical analysis to describe the relationship between the information available and the judgement or decisions made.

Another advantage of judgement analysis relates to the scale of the studies that can be undertaken. Whereas process-tracing studies use comparatively few, carefully selected clinical scenarios, judgement analysis can examine a large number of decision-makers' policies on a wide range of decisions. Therefore, although judgement analysis produces a paramorphic (symbolic) rather than an isomorphic (exact) representation of the decision process, generalisations of policy use can be made.

A study by Kirwan *et al.* (1986) confirmed the superiority of the judgement analysis approach in researching clinical decision making. They examined the policies of 89 rheumatologists in prescribing anti-inflammatory medication. As the rheumatologists saw patients, they were asked to record levels of five types of cue (pieces of information) such as degree of early morning stiffness for each patient. They were also asked to record their decision for each patient in terms of the level of medication they then prescribed. These data were analysed to identify the prescribing policies they were using in their practice. The doctors were then asked to explain how they assessed this type of patient, in order to simulate how they taught their stated policies to medical students. The prescribing policies that they were found to have used in practice were compared with the policies that they thought they had used (stated policies). Their stated policies were found to be a poor predictor of their actual policies ($R^2 = 34\%$).

The cue information recorded from this study was used to create a set of 50 paper patients (including a replicate set of 20 to test for test-retest reliability). The rheumatologists then prescribed for the paper patients and the results were examined. The judgements over paper patients were found to correlate well with those over real patients ($R^2 = 88\%$). However the stated prescribing policies of the doctors were again poor predictors of actual policies used ($R^2 = 39\%$). One explanation for this is that some unconscious processing had occurred so that clinicians were not able to accurately describe their practice policies. The more experienced the participants were, the less able they were to say what they knew (Hoffman, 1987; Nisbett and Wilson, 1977). It is important, therefore, that methods of research into clinical judgement avoid relying on the verbalisation of participants. Judgement analysis can find out not only what cues are used in decision making but also the weighting and combination of these cues. In addition, statistically identified policies can be compared with participants' subjective policies (how they think they have made their judgements) to identify individuals' level of self-insight as to their own policy.

This is a potentially valuable methodology but it has rarely been used with occupational therapists until now and its potential has not been fully exploited (Harries and Gilhooly, 2003a; Unsworth *et al.*, 1997). The next section examines experts' thinking strategies, insight and how feedback can be used to teach professional decision-making policies.

Expertise development, self-insight and feedback

The pattern recognition and heuristics of the intuitive mode of thinking can only be used when previous experience is available to the decision maker. This means that the mode of thought used is influenced by the experience of the decision maker and, hence, their level of expertise. Analytical processing has to be used when the person is less practised in a cognitive task, but intuitive strategies are used when he is more practised in a reasoning task and the information is familiar (Benner, 1984; Elstein *et al.*, 1990; Norman *et al.*, 1992).

Task characteristics, such as stability and availability of task information, are also thought to have a strong influence on the type of cognitive processing used (Shanteau, 1992). Different types of reasoning task, involving different content, have different task characteristics and are associated with different modes of cognition. The mode used is, therefore, a result of the combined effect of the practitioner's level of experience and the task characteristics.

For example, Roberts (1996) demonstrated that the type of reasoning used by occupational therapists varies according to the level of expertise and the nature of the task. In her research, 38 practitioners wrote down their thoughts immediately after reading three referral letters. Some practitioners initially used rapid formulations of the issues involved (pattern matchers/heuristic reasoners). They mentioned their recognition of the scenario and recalled previous cases. Other practitioners searched for cues and reasoned using various hypotheses, sometimes not reaching any specific formulation. The latter group appeared to have less experience on which to draw. The rapid formulators did not show intuitive reasoning exclusively but used hypothetico-deductive reasoning when considering some aspects of the case. In these instances, it appeared that participants were less familiar with the information.

Hypothetico-deductive reasoning is more accessible than intuitive thought, as it involves more conscious thinking. Elstein *et al.* (1978) identified hypothetico-deductive reasoning as the strategy for diagnosis formation in medicine. Occupational therapists also looked for, and found, hypothetico-deductive reasoning in diagnosis of occupational dysfunction (Fleming, 1991a). However, when later clinical research was conducted within the specific task of diagnosis formation, it was found that other forms of thinking also occur. These are apparent when comparing differences between the reasoning strategies of novices and experienced practitioners (Elstein *et al.*, 1990). Schmidt *et al.* (1990) found that experts in familiar situations do not usually display explicit hypothesis testing but, when confronted with a familiar problem, use a rapid and automatic form of processing that is acknowledged as intuitive reasoning. Having the advantage of previous experience, they have developed a store of 'scripts' and use pattern matching to trigger the direct automatic retrieval of an appropriate script (Abernathy and Hamm, 1994).

Early research into clinical reasoning used mainly qualitative methodologies, such as process tracing and ethnographic approaches. The first medical study, conducted by Elstein *et al.* (1978), used process tracing to analyse the verbal protocols of clinicians. Roberts (1996) and Munroe (1996) conducted the first large studies on occupational therapists' reasoning processes, using a process-tracing approach and an ethnographic approach respectively. Ethnographic techniques are derived from anthropological approaches that value participant observation and in-depth interviewing. The AOTA/AOTF study (Mattingly and Fleming, 1994), the first large study of the reasoning of American occupational therapists, also used an ethnographic approach. In these early studies, intuitive reasoning was not given much attention. For example, in the AOTA/AOTF study, intuitive reasoning was only nominally identified and was described as difficult to map (Fleming, 1991b), but no details were given of the ways in which mapping was attempted.

The ethnographic and information-processing methods appear to have had little success in establishing the thoughts used in clinicians' intuitive thinking. These methods rely heavily on the reasoner's awareness of how they are using information to make judgements, and they are limited in their ability to access the more unconscious, rapid and unrecoverable reasoning at the intuitive end of the continuum (Ericsson and Simon, 1980).

The efficacy of using verbal reports to access thinking has been drawn into question as being inefficient and misrepresentative, particularly with regard to accessing the thinking of experts (Hoffman, 1987). Concurrent verbalisations, at best, can only access the content of working memory or the information attended to (but not necessarily how it is used), and retrospective verbalisations are prone to forgetting and post-hoc rationalisation (Ericsson and Simon, 1980). If intuitive thought is non-recoverable, the access of decision makers into their thinking must be reflected in their levels of self-insight (Ericsson and Simon, 1980; Nisbett and Wilson, 1977).

Self-insight

In the 1970s, researchers turned their attention to studying self-insight. Self-insight, in this context, can be defined as the knowledge of, and ability to describe, one's own decision-making policies (Harries et al., 2000).

To identify levels of self-insight, early research compared how decision makers thought they had used information (cue weights) with how they had actually used it. This was most commonly done by comparing subjective weights with statistical weights derived from regression analysis, or by comparing R^2 values derived from predictions with subjective weights with R^2 values derived from regression weights. Results generally showed that insight was poor (Brehmer and Brehmer, 1988) and that decision makers usually overestimated the number and importance of cues (Elstein et al., 1978). It was found that the development of expertise tends to lessen rather than improve self-insight (Slovic and Lichenstein, 1971).

Occupational therapists in the UK have been trying to gain insight into the different types of thinking that they use, as part of a wider attempt to make professional reasoning explicit, although no formal study had been conducted at this time. Donald Schön (1983) advocated reflection-in-action as a means of developing awareness of the intuitive, tacit type of thinking which governs everyday practice. His ideas have been warmly welcomed by the occupational therapy profession and have been incorporated into the clinical supervision of qualified practitioners as well as the clinical education of occupational therapy students (Brunel University, 1999). However, there is evidence that challenges the value of such introspection or reflection on cognitive processes. I decided to undertake an empirical investigation into occupational therapists' capacity to accurately report their judgements.

The self-insight of the occupational therapists participating in the referral prioritisation policy study was investigated by collecting data on their stated policies via a questionnaire and comparing them with the tacit policies identified through the judgement analysis study. Individual participants were asked to rate each cue between 0 and 10 to represent the influence that that cue had on their prioritisation of the referral (while assuming that the values of the other cues are held constant). A score of 0 was used to indicate that the information had no influence on the judgement. A score of 10 indicated that the information had a maximum bearing on the judgement.

The actual policies that were used in practice had already been calculated from the ratings each participant gave to the 90 referrals (Harries and Gilhooly, 2003a). These represented each individual's objective weights as opposed to the subjective weights.

Both these sets of data could then be correlated to identify the level of self-insight of the participants. A good match would indicate a good level of self-insight.

The results showed that although the self-insight of the group was fair ($r = 0.605$, df = 39, $N = 40$) the range of self-insight varied greatly among the participants (range 0.081 to 0.862). This wide range of values suggests that it is not only the type of task that influences self-insight but also the capacity of the individual. The results demonstrated that insight was greatest for the most and least important cues, while the influence of those cues that were not given very high or very low importance was generally overestimated. This phenomenon pertaining to the middle ground has been recognised since the early clinical studies in decision making (Elstein *et al.*, 1978).

Some participants had poor self-insight scores. They may have been the least able of the participants, since Kruger and Dunning (1999) have shown that those who have less ability often have less self-insight. Conversely, they may have been those with the most ability, since poor self-insight can indicate that expert intuitive thinking, which is not easily accessible, is being used (McMackin and Slovic, 2000).

As some occupational therapists have been found to have limited self-insight, it may be a little unrealistic to presume that reflective practice has certain benefits. If self-insight is less than optimal, reflection can lead the individual to focus on inappropriate information, thus leading to a deterioration of subsequent decisions (Wilson and Schooler, 1991). Reflective practice may be most valuable for novice therapists who are using analytical thinking, or for those following explicit team policy. For intuitive thinkers, reflective practice needs to be focused on the information that is actually used in their decision making rather than on that which is not.

One essential reason for establishing the policies of our clinical experts is to ensure that education is truly evidence-based. Reliable and valid knowledge of how the profession's experts identify and use information can be gathered to train students in good decision making.

Training novices with expert policy

In 2003, the referral prioritisation policies modelled by the satisfied specialists (Harries and Gilhooly, 2003b) were taught to third-year undergraduate occupational therapy students (Weiss *et al.*, 2006). The aim was to investigate whether the students could use the policies of the expert occupational therapists. A one-group pre-test, post-test design was chosen to measure any effects of training. Students were asked to give priority ratings (dependent variables) to occupational therapy referrals before and after training (feedforward phase). The presence of the training information represented the independent variable.

The students were presented with a set of 90 referrals identical to those used with the expert group, in order to facilitate direct comparison between expert and novice prioritisation ratings. If, following training, the students' prioritisation ratings became more like the experts', then the training would have had its desired effect. The referrals were divided into two sets to provide a pre- and post- set for the students (Cooksey, 1996). A total of 52 referrals were used before training to establish the students' initial judgement policies. A total of 38 referrals were used after training to test how well the students had been able to use the expert policies. In order to analyse consistency of policy application, 22 replicates of the pre-training referrals were added to the end of the pre-training set and 10 replicates of the post-training referrals were added to the end of the post-training set.

Training information should comprise task information as opposed to cognitive information (Balzer et al., 1989; Balzer and Sulsky, 1992; Hammond and Summers, 1972). Cue weight policy is one type of task information needed to make the desired decisions, in this case, to prioritise a referral effectively. The optimal cue weights used by one subgroup of occupational therapists, the satisfied specialists ($N = 9$), was identified as the cue weight policy needed to train the judgements of novices. The experts used three cues: reason for referral, diagnosis and level of violence. These cue weights were presented to the students as bar charts, informing them which cues they should pay attention to and to what degree. For example, the reason for referral cue gave a very high rating to physical and psychological needs while monitoring of new medication was given a very low rating. In order to promote understanding of why the experts had used their policies, and to assist in memorising quantitative data, descriptive information was also provided. This identified the clinical reasoning that supported experts' prioritisation policies.

By using the training information, students were then able to rate the referrals more like the experts, indicating improvements in knowledge and cognitive control. Students' weighting policies improved with training so that their prioritisation judgements were much more like the experts, but in addition they used fewer cues, a skill that has been shown to be a clear sign of expertise (Shanteau et al., 1991; Stewart et al., 1992). This training package has now been made into a freely available web training tool and is being used by occupational therapists and by universities as an educational tool (Harries, 2006).

Conclusion

At the start of this chapter I posed some questions: how do we make wise clinical judgements, how much insight do we have into our judgements, how capable are we of reflection, which policies should we be teaching novices and how can we teach expert thinking? I feel I have begun to understand some of the issues involved in answering these questions.

Identifying what is a wise judgement is a hard task but it is key to clinical reasoning research. I have tried using issues of group consensus, consistency of policy use and coherence to current professional recommendations. These are not foolproof: experts may agree but who is to say they are correct; experts may be consistent but they may be consistently wrong and political trends can change with the wind. My recent research continues to examine how best to identify wise decisions (Weiss *et al.*, 2006).

I do not feel we have full insight into our reasoning. Intuitive strategies can cause some thoughts to become subconscious and we certainly cannot reflect on that which we cannot access. We appear to be able to identify what information is most important to our decisions and what information is least important. However we also tend to overestimate the importance and amount of information we use. How then, in verbal reports, can we separate what is the wood from the trees?

To make our thinking explicit, the study of clinical judgement needs to use a wide range of research methods. It is the triangulation of information from these research methodologies that can bring us nearer to understanding our thinking processes. The qualitative methodologies are well suited to identifying the factors needed to make the judgements, as well as the context for the decision making itself. Some of the quantitative methods, such as judgement analysis, can then be used to model how information can be weighted and combined to come to a particular decision.

Modelled policies offer one avenue to investigate how we utilise information to make decisions. If novices can follow them they can be used to change individuals' methods of thinking. My research has shown that this is possible. The key is to find the policies that we want them to use.

The novices who learnt the modelled prioritisation policy have to be admired. They were able to change the way they used information and adapt to the experienced therapists' way of working. It is not easy to change how we think: we need to remain open and receptive to new research methods and new findings so we can continue to grow in our understanding of our thinking processes.

Note

Visual Basic programming was carried out by Dr Clare Harries, Research Fellow, Department of Psychology, University College London.

References

Abernathy, C.M. and Hamm, R.M. (1994) *Surgical Scripts: Master Surgeons Think Aloud about 43 Common Surgical Problems*, Hanley and Belfus, Philadephia.

Alvervik, A. and Sviden, G. (1996) On clinical reasoning: patterns of reflection on practice. *Occupational Therapy Journal of Research.* **16**(2): 98–110.

Arkes, H.A. and Hammond, K.R. (1986) *Judgement and decision making*, Cambridge University Press, Cambridge, UK.

Bailey, D. (1990) Reasons for attrition from occupational therapy. *American Journal of Occupational Therapy*, **44**, 23–9.

Balzer, W. and Sulsky, L. (1992) Task information, cognitive information, or functional validity information: which components of cognitive feedback affect performance? *Organizational Behavior and Human Decision Processes*, **53**, 35–54.

Balzer, W.K., Doherty, M.E. and O'Connor, R. (1989) Effects of cognitive feedback on performance. *Psychological Bulletin*, **106**(3), 410–33.

Bassett, H. and Lloyd, C. (2001) Occupational therapy in mental health: managing stress and burnout. *British Journal of Occupational Therapy*, **64**(8), 406–11.

Benner, P. (1984) *From Novice to Expert: Excellence and Power in Clinical Nursing Practice*, Addison-Wesley, Menlo Park, CA.

Brehmer, A. and Brehmer, B. (1988) What have we learnt about human judgement from thirty years of policy capturing? in *Human Judgement: The SJT View* (eds B. Brehmer and C. Joyce), North Holland, Elsevier Science.

Brunel University (1999) *BSc (Hons) Occupational Therapy: student course handbook*, Department of Health and Social Care, Brunel University, London.

Brunswik, E. (1952) The conceptual framework of psychology. *International Encyclopedia of Unified Science*, University of Chicago Press, Chicago, **1**(10), 1–102.

Cooksey, R.W. (1996) *Judgement analysis: theory, methods and applications*, Academic Press, London.

Corrigan, K. (2002) CMHT's: embedding the occupational perspective. *British Journal of Occupational Therapy*, **65**(2), 100.

Craik, C., Austin, C., Chacksfield, J.D., Richards, G. and Schell, D. (1998a) College of Occupational Therapists: position paper on the way ahead for research, education and practice in mental health. *British Journal of Occupational Therapy*, **61**(9), 390–2.

Craik, C., Chacksfield, J. and Richards, G. (1998b) A survey of occupational therapy practitioners in mental health. *British Journal of Occupational Therapy*, **61**, 227–34.

Craik, C., Austin, C. and Schell, D. (1999) A national survey of occupational therapy managers in mental health. *British Journal of Occupational Therapy*, **62**(5), 220–8.

Creek, J. (1990) *Occupational Therapy and Mental Health*, Churchill Livingstone, Edinburgh.

Dawson, N.V. (1987) Systematic errors in medical decision making. *Journal of General Internal Medicine*, **2**(May/June), 183–7.

Dawson, N.V. (1993) Physician judgement in clinical settings: methodological influences and cognitive performance. *Clinical Chemistry*, **39**(7), 1468–80.

Dawson, N.V. and Cebul, R.C. (1990) Advances in quantitative techniques for making medical decisions: the last decade. *Evaluation in the Health Professions*, **13**(1), 37–62.

Department of Health (1983) *The Mental Health Act*, HMSO, London.

Department of Health (1995) *Building Bridges: A Guide to Inter-agency Working for the Care and Protection of Severely Mentally Ill People*, HMSO, London.

Department of Health (1999) *National Service Framework for Mental Health*, HMSO, London.

Department of Health (2000) *The NHS Plan*. National Health Service, London.

Doherty, M.E. and Kurz, E.M. (1996) Social judgement theory. *Thinking and Reasoning*, **2**(2/3), 109–40.

Elstein, A. (1976) Clinical judgement: psychological research and medical practice. *Science*, **194**, 696–700.

Elstein, A.E. and Schwartz, A. (2000) Clinical reasoning in medicine, in *Clinical Reasoning in the Health Professions* (eds J. Higgs and M. Jones), Butterworth-Heinemann, Oxford.

Elstein, A.S., Shulman, L.S. and Sprafka, S.A. (1978) *Medical Problem Solving: An Analysis of Clinical Reasoning*, Harvard University Press, Cambridge, MA.

Elstein, A.S., Shulman, L.S. and Sprafka, S.A. (1990) Medical problem solving: a ten year retrospective. *Evaluation and the Health Professions*, **13**(1), 5–36.

Ericsson, K.A. and Simon, H.A. (1980) Verbal reports as data. *Psychological Review*, **87**(3), 215–51.

Fleming, M.H. (1991a) Clinical reasoning in medicine compared with clinical reasoning in occupational therapy. *American Journal of Occupational Therapy*, **45**(11), 988–96.

Fleming, M.H. (1991b) The therapist with the three-track mind. *American Journal of Occupational Therapy*, **45**(11), 1007–14.

Forsyth, K. and Summerfield Mann, L. (2002) Generic working. *British Journal of Occupational Therapy*, **65**(6), 296–7.

Fortune, T. and Ryan, S. (1996) Applying clinical reasoning: a caseload management system for community occupational therapists. *British Journal of Occupational Therapists*, **59**(5), 207–11.

Fossie, E. (1996) Using the occupational performance history interview (OPHI): therapists' reflections. *British Journal of Occupational Therapy*, **59**(5), 223–8.

Fox, J. and Alvey, P. (1983) ABC of computing. *British Medical Journal*, **287**(10 Sept.), 742–6.

Fryback, D. (1983) *Decision Maker, Quantify Thyself!* 5th Annual Meeting of the Society for Medical Decision Makers, Toronto, Canada.

Gordon, C. (1991) Supporting acts. *The British Journal of Healthcare Computing*, September: 29–30.

Grime, H. (1990) Receiving referrals: decision making by the community occupational therapist. *British Journal of Occupational Therapy*, **53**(2), 53–6.

Hagedorn, R. (1996) Clinical decision making in familiar cases: a model of the process and implications for practice. *British Journal of Occupational Therapy*, **59**(5), 217–22.

Hammond, K.R. and Summers, D.A. (1972) Cognitive control. *Psychological Review*, **79**(1), 58–67.

Hammond, K., Stewart, T., Brehmer, B. and Steinmann, D. (1975) Social judgement theory: applications in policy formation, in *Human Judgement and Decision Processes* (eds M. Kaplan and S. Schwartz), Academic Press, San Diego, CA, pp. 271–312.

Harries, C. (1995) Judgement analysis of patient management: general practitioners' policies and self-insight (PhD thesis), University of Plymouth, Plymouth, UK.

Harries, C., Evans, J. StB. T. and Dennis, I. (2000) Measuring doctors' self-insight into their prescribing decisions. *Applied Cognitive Psychology*, **14**, 455–77.

Harries, P. (2006) Editorial: The development of a web-based tool for training referral prioritization skills. *International Journal of Therapy and Rehabilitation*, **13**(6).

Harries, P.A. (1996a) A study to identify, in the field of mental health, the factors influencing occupational therapists' decision making as to whether or not to accept a referral, University of Exeter, Exeter, UK.

Harries, P.A. (1996b) *Naming and framing occupational therapy practice in community mental health work*. Vth European Congress of Occupational Therapy, Madrid.

Harries, P.A. (1998) A study to identify, in the field of community mental health, the factors influencing OTs' decision making as to whether or not to accept a referral. *British Journal of Occupational Therapists*, **61**(4), 156.

Harries, P.A. (2002) CMHT's: specialist versus generalist roles. *British Journal of Occupational Therapy*, **65**(1), 40–1.

Harries, P.A. and Gilhooly, K. (2003a) Identifying occupational therapists' referral priorities in community health. *Occupational Therapy International*, **10**(2), 150–64.

Harries, P. and Gilhooly, K. (2003b) Generic and specialist occupational therapy casework in community mental health. *British Journal of Occupational Therapy*, **66**(3): 101–9.

Hershey, J.C. and Baron, J. (1987) Clinical reasoning and cognitive processes. *Medical Decision Making*, **7**(4), 203–11.

Hoffman, R.R. (1987) The problem of extracting the knowledge of experts from the perspective of experimental psychology. *AI Magazine*, 53–67.

Hoffrage, U., Lindsey, S., Hertwig, R. and Gigerenzer, G. (2000) Communicating statistical information. *Science*, **290**(5500), 2261–2.

Job, T. (1996) A system for determining the priority of referrals within a multidisciplinary community mental health team. *British Journal of Occupational Therapy*, **62**(11), 486–90.

Kirwan, J.R., Chaput de Saintonge, D.M., Joyce, C.R., Holmes, J. and Currey, H.L. (1986) Inability of rheumatologists to describe their true policies for assessing rheumatoid arthritis. *Annals of Rheumatic Diseases*, **45**(2), 156–61.

Kruger, J. and Dunning, D. (1999) Unskilled and unaware of it: how difficulties in recognizing one's own incompetence lead to inflated self-assessments. *Journal of Personality & Social Psychology*, **77**(6), 1121–34.

Lloyd-Smith, W. (1997) Evidence-based practice and occupational therapy. *British Journal of Occupational Therapy*, **60**(11), 474–8.

Mattingly, C. (1991) The narrative nature of clinical reasoning. *American Journal of Occupational Therapy*, **45**(11), 998–1005.

Mattingly, C. and Fleming, M.H. (1994) *Clinical Reasoning: Forms of Inquiry in a Therapeutic Practice*, F.A. Davis Co., Philadephia.

McMackin, J. and Slovic, P. (2000) When does explicit justification impair decision making? *Applied Cognitive Psychology*, **14**, 527–41.

Meehl, P. (1954) *Clinical versus statistical prediction: A theoretical analysis and a review of the evidence*, University of Minneapolis, Minneapolis, MI.

Munroe, H. (1996) Clinical reasoning in community occupational therapy. *British Journal of Occupational Therapy*, **59**(5), 196–202.

Newell, A. and Simon, H. (1972) *Human Problem Solving*, Prentice Hall, Englewood Cliffs, NJ.

Nisbett, R. and Wilson, T. (1977) Telling more than we can know: verbal reports on mental processes. *Psychological Review*, **84**, 231–59.

Norman, G.R. and Schmidt, H.G. (1992) The psychological basis of problem-based learning: a review of the evidence. *Academic Medicine*, **67**(9), 557–65.

Parker, H. (2001) The role of occupational therapists in community mental health teams. *British Journal of Occupational Therapy*, **64**(12), 609–11.

Reed, K. and Sanderson, S. (1992) *Concepts of Occupational Therapy*, Wilkins & Wilkins, Baltimore, MD.

Roberts, A.E. (1996) Approaches to reasoning in occupational therapy: a critical exploration. *British Journal of Occupational Therapy*, **59**(5), 233–6.

Ryan, S. (1990) *Clinical Reasoning: A Descriptive Study Comparing Novice and Experienced Occupational Therapists*, Columbia University, New York.

Savage, L.J. (1954) *The Foundations of Statistics*, John Wiley & Sons, New York.

Schmidt, H.G., Norman, G.R. and Boshuizen, H.P.A. (1990) A cognitive perspective on medical expertise: theory and implications. *Academic Medicine*, **65**, 611–21.

Schön, D. (1983) *The Reflective Practitioner: How Professionals Think in Action*, Basic Books, New York.

Shanteau, J. (1992) Competence in experts: the role of task characteristics. *Organizational Behavior and Human Decision Processes*, **53**, 252–66.

Shanteau, J. (2001) Evaluating expertise. *The Brunswik Society Newsletter.* October, p. 16.

Shanteau, J., Grier, M. and Berner, E. (1991) Teaching decision making skills to student nurses, in *Teaching Decision Making to Adolescents* (ed. J.B.V. Brown), Lawrence Erlbaum Associates, Hillsdale, NJ, pp. 185–206.

Slovic, P. and Lichenstein, S. (1971) Comparison of Bayesian and regression approaches to the study of information processing in judgement. *Organizational Behavior and Human Performance*, **6**, 649–744.

Spalding, N. (1999) The assessment of surgical priority of occupational therapists. *British Journal of Occupational Therapy*, **62**(5), 229–31.

Stewart, T., Heideman, K., Moninger, W. and Reagan-Cirincione, P. (1992) Effects of improved information on the components of skill in weather forecasting. *Organizational Behavior and Human Decision Processes*, **53**, 107–34.

Sturgess, J. and Poulsen, A. (1983) The prevalence of burnout in occupational therapists. *Occupational Therapy in Mental Health*, **3**, 47–60.

Tape, T.G., Heckerling, P.S., Ornato, J.P. and Wigton, R.S. (1991) Use of clinical judgment analysis to explain regional variations in physicians' accuracies in diagnosing pneumonia. *Medical Decision Making*, **11**, 189–97.

Tversky, A. and Kahneman, D. (1981) The framing of decisions and the psychology of choice. *Science*, **211**, 453–8.

Unsworth, C.A., Thomas, S.A. and Greenwood, K.M. (1997) Decision polarization among rehabilitation team recommendations concerning discharge housing for stroke patients. *International Journal of Rehabilitation Research*, **20**, 51–69.

Weiss, D.J., Shanteau, J. and Harries, P. (2006) People who judge people. *Journal of Behavioral Decision Making*, **19**, 441–54.

Wilson, T. and Schooler, J. (1991) Thinking too much: introspection can reduce the quality of preferences and decisions. *Journal of Personality and Social Psychology*, **60**, 181–92.

Making sense of research utilisation

10

Katrina Bannigan

Introduction

Evidence-based practice has become a key feature of modern health and social services. It 'requires that decisions about health [and social] care are based on the best available, current, valid and relevant evidence. These decisions should be made by those receiving care, informed by the tacit and explicit knowledge of those providing care, within the context of available resources' (Dawes *et al.*, 2005: 4). There is a clear expectation that occupational therapists will be evidence-based practitioners (Department of Health, n.d.; College of Occupational Therapists, 2005; Ilott and White, 2001) and, while occupational therapists are enthusiastic about evidence-based practice (Upton, 1999), as with other professionals working in health and social care, there is a gap between their enthusiasm and action (Grimshaw and Thomson, 1998). That occupational therapists are unable to translate their evident enthusiasm into action suggests that evidence-based practice may not be easy for them. The difficulty is that evidence-based practice requires an ability to use research findings, so the problem is the research–practice gap. The research–practice gap reflects a myth among professionals working in health and social care; when asked, they state that research findings are used to underpin their practice when in reality they are not (Kirk, 1998). Anecdotally, it is estimated that there is a seven- to ten-year time lag between the publication of research findings and their use in practice.

It appears that the research–practice gap exists for occupational therapists because they perceive and/or experience barriers to research utilisation (Closs and Lewin, 1998; Metcalfe *et al.*, 2001; Pollock *et al.*, 2000). Research utilisation involves the application of the findings of research to practice. A barrier to research utilisation is 'anything that interferes with research utilisation, or is perceived as an interference' (Linde, 1989, p. 18). The range of barriers perceived and/or experienced by occupational therapists suggests that research utilisation is a complex problem. For example, therapists find that there is insufficient time to implement new ideas, no time to read research, statistical analyses are not understandable, literature is not compiled in one place, literature reports conflicting results and it is not easy to transfer findings into daily practice (Closs and Lewin, 1998; Metcalfe *et al.*, 2001; Pollock *et al.*, 2000).

This chapter will:

- explore the disputed nature of research utilisation;
- look at what is involved in research utilisation;
- consider how the use of research findings can be fostered; and
- draw on systems thinking to explore a way forward for thinking about and researching research utilisation.

This will provide an indication of the issues that need to be addressed in order to turn occupational therapists' evident enthusiasm for research into the regular application of research findings in everyday practice.

The disputed nature of research utilisation

The study of research utilisation is a nascent field in which there is no widely accepted definition of research utilisation or other key concepts (Crosswaite and Curtice, 1994). There are also a number of synonymous or interchangeable terms in use, such as clinical effectiveness, evidence-based practice, innovation diffusion, research uptake, technology transfer and utilisation, but it is not always clear whether the words are being used in the same or different ways. This variety of terms also makes the literature difficult to locate. There appear to be two reasons why a lack of clarity exists around the subject. First, research utilisation is a part of the wider concept of evidence-based practice and, second, research utilisation is a generic skill.

Evidence-based practice and research utilisation

Evidence-based practice has been described as 'a process of turning clinicians' problems into questions and then systematically locating, appraising, and using contemporaneous research findings as the basis for clinical decisions' (Rosenberg and Donald, 1995, p. 1122). This makes this process analogous to research utilisation. Research utilisation is a process in which decisions are made about whether or not research findings are generally applicable to practice.

In evidence-based practice, any general decisions made about research use are balanced against service users' values, clinical judgement and a consideration of resources in the specific instance. For example, research may indicate that occupational therapy can help people with rheumatoid arthritis to do daily chores such as dressing, cooking and cleaning and with less pain, particularly if the intervention includes training, advice, counselling and advice on joint protection (Steultjens *et al.*, 2004). However, if an occupational therapist is working with an individual who has rheumatoid arthritis and the individual had no interest in learning about joint protection to facilitate their activities of daily living, it would not be appropriate to provide this intervention even though research indicates that it is an effective intervention to use. (Obviously the reasoning underpinning this decision would have to be explicitly documented in the individual's notes.)

Rosenberg and Donald (1995) identified four key components of evidence-based practice: formulating a clear clinical question from a patient's problem; searching the literature for relevant clinical articles; evaluating (critically appraising) the evidence for its validity and usefulness, and implementing useful findings in clinical practice. Sackett *et al.* (1997, 2000) and Straus *et al.* (2005) extended this schema by adding a fifth component:

1. Converting information needs into answerable questions;
2. Tracking down, with maximum efficiency, the best evidence with which to answer them;
3. Critically appraising that evidence for its validity (closeness to the truth) and usefulness (clinical applicability);
4. Applying the results of this appraisal in our clinical practice; and
5. Evaluating our performance (p. 3).

Evidence-based practice has been widely adopted in health and social care, including the allied health professions (Enderby *et al.*, 1998). 'To give you some evidence of the impressive take-up of this concept, there is a very long list of journal articles within *Index Medicus* that have incorporated the term evidence-based in their title over the last eight years' (Sutherland, 2001, p. 3). Recently, a consensus statement was published: the *Sicily statement on evidence-based practice* (Dawes *et al.*, 2005). It clearly located the use of research findings in the context of decisions about health and social care: these decisions include those receiving care; they are informed by the tacit and explicit knowledge of those providing care, and they are made within the context of available resources. This shows that the concept of evidence-based practice has evolved in the last decade. Research use is now recognised as only one feature of evidence-based practice, alongside service user values, clinical judgement and a consideration of resources.

Defining research utilisation

Many of the issues faced by occupational therapists are similar to those faced by other professionals working in health and social care. For example, barriers (whether real or perceived) are a reality for most professional groups when trying to increase the use of research findings. This is because, like communication and record keeping, research utilisation is a generic skill. It is accepted that there are differences between professional groups but there seem to be more similarities than differences, and a focus on the similarities initially may be more useful than a focus on the differences. The emphasis in *The NHS Plan* (Department of Health, 2000), and subsequent policy, on interdisciplinary working suggests that working across boundaries is not natural for professionals working in health and social care; why else would a policy directive be needed to make it happen? Many probably chose to work in a profession in the first place because they want to work with like-minded people focused on a particular aspect of health and social care work. In relation to research utilisation, this has resulted in an 'invisible college' of researchers (Rogers, 1995) and a body of research that is difficult to locate.

Perhaps if research utilisation were tackled across professional boundaries there would be more coherence in the research conducted, less duplication of effort and a critical mass of researchers working on this topic. This is because the individuals or small groups currently spread across different professions could pool their efforts to develop research programmes that move forward the understanding of the subject. Moving this field of research on from a disparate and invisible college (Rogers, 1995) to a recognised field of research may help practitioners such as occupational therapists to locate information about research utilisation more easily. It would also mean that coherence in the field would be increased because key terms would have to be defined so that there could be more comparison between studies. The current 'terminological tangle' (Larsen, 1980), cited in Estabrooks, 1997) is not acceptable where:

> Definitions are frequently missing or absent from articles, different disciplines use different terminology, most of the literature rests on assumptions that are rarely made explicit, and investigators, at least in nursing, appear to have assumed that terminology and concepts from other disciplines are readily transferable to nursing.
>
> (Estabrooks, 1997, p. 6)

The disparate nature of the field may partly explain why a gap exists between the enthusiasm and action of occupational therapists when it comes to using research findings; after all, if literature on the subject cannot be found, practitioners cannot use it. Equally, if research utilisation has eluded a standard definition and our understanding has been evolving, it is perhaps not surprising that therapists are enthusiastic about it but find it difficult to operationalise in their everyday practice. The implication of this analysis is that, as occupational therapists, we need to recognise research utilisation (and evidence-based practice) as a generic skill. We will then focus on research utilisation and evidence-based practice per se rather than on research use in occupational therapy or evidence-based occupational therapy specifically, which perpetuate the current state of affairs.

There have been many attempts to define research utilisation, but McCurren (1995) offered a definition which recognised that research utilisation may involve verification rather than change, and this definition therefore may be the most fitting: 'a process in which the products of research are applied to verify current practice or to change current practice' (p. 132). The emphasis on verification is important because, contrary to the usual assumption, research findings will sometimes verify current practice rather than highlight the need to change practice. However, this definition does need to be slightly modified by inclusion of the word *valid*, to signal that research utilisation involves a process of identifying whether the research findings (the products) are valid: 'a process in which the [valid] products of research are applied to verify current practice or to change current practice'. This is important because only current, valid and relevant findings should be applied to practice (Dawes *et al.*, 2005). It is only once a decision has been made about the rigour of the research findings that they should be compared to current practice to assess whether practice needs to be changed or not. This modified definition indicates that:

- research utilisation involves a process;
- part of the process involves making judgements about the rigour of research;
- another part of the process involves making a decision about whether these findings verify or need to be applied to practice; and
- sometimes, but not always, change will be involved.

Research utilisation is a macro skill that is a composite of a number of other sub- or micro skills. However, it has been suggested that definitions of research utilisation, like McCurren's (1995), define only one form of research utilisation, that is, instrumental use. This understanding of research use will be discussed before the suppositions underpinning McCurren's (1995) definition are explored in more detail.

Forms of research utilisation

Research utilisation as a concept can be differentiated into different forms. In applying work from other fields to nursing, Stetler (1994) suggested that research utilisation can be understood as instrumental, conceptual or symbolic use of research based knowledge:

- Instrumental use is the 'concrete application of knowledge; including research . . . direct development of policies, procedures or standards is one such instrumental use' (Stetler, 1994, pp. 16–17).

- Conceptual use 'refers to cognitive application and is best embodied through the term enlightenment, in which utilisation changes understanding or the way one thinks about a situation . . . This type of use may occur more frequently than the concrete application of findings, and the related gradual, cumulative understanding of a topic may lead to changes in behaviour that are less specific and not easy to pinpoint in time' (Stetler, 1994, p. 17).

- Symbolic use is where 'information is used to legitimate a policy or a currently held position' (Stetler, 1994, p. 17).

While this conceptualisation was developed in the United States and, as Estabrooks (1997) observed, 'has largely not been followed through in the nursing literature' (pp. 19–20) it has an inherent logic for those working in the field of research utilisation in the United Kingdom. For example, Closs and Cheater (1994) and Carter (1996) have both discussed this conceptualisation and concluded that the ideas translate to the UK context.

Estabrooks (1997) examined this conceptualisation in more detail. She conducted a study with the aim of increasinging 'existing knowledge of research utilisation in nursing by expanding our understanding of the causal mechanisms underlying the utilisation and non-utilisation of research by nurses' (Estabrooks, 1997, p. 4). The model tested was that 'overall research utilisation is made up of (caused by) instrumental, conceptual and symbolic utilisation' (Estabrooks, 1997, p. 40). Estabrooks augmented the definitions of the terms:

- Instrumental utilisation: a concrete application of research where the research is normally translated (on an organisational or nursing unit level) into a material and useable form such as a clinical protocol, a clinical decision algorithm, or the currently popular clinical practice guidelines. At the individual level the research may be applied 'directly' as an intervention without translation into another form such as a protocol. It may be applied fully, partially, or in modified form. The research in this is used to make specific decisions/interventions, i.e., to direct practice in a tangible and measurable way.

- Conceptual utilisation: the use of research such that the research changes one's thinking but not necessarily one's particular action. In this case, the research informs and enlightens the decision-maker (nurse), influencing decisions and interventions in less tangible ways than instrumental utilisation.

- Symbolic (or political) utilisation: the use of research as a persuasive or political tool to legitimate a position or practice. It is commonly used to influence colleagues and decision makers at local, regional, and/or higher levels of authority.

(Estabrooks, 1997, p. 42)

She also changed the labels from instrumental, conceptual and symbolic to direct, indirect and persuasive, respectively (Estabrooks, 1997). This was because she thought that these words were more readily understood, and less cumbersome, for both researchers and practitioners. In her study she found 'no indication that the respondents had difficulty differentiating between direct, indirect and persuasive research utilisation' (Estabrooks, 1997, p. 125). She also noted that 'It is apparent that there is not one "grand" or integrating theory of innovation diffusion or research utilisation' (Estabrooks, 1997, p. 36). She went on to develop 'a model of research utilisation that illustrates the causal influence of direct (instrumental), indirect (conceptual) and persuasive (symbolic) research utilisation on overall research utilisation' (Estabrooks, 1997, abstract).

While there were some limitations to Estabrooks' study, for example, a low response rate, the model she developed appears to be useful as a model of research utilisation in nursing. Despite the fact that the theoretical development and empirical testing has only been conducted in nursing, it also makes sense that research use will be direct, indirect and persuasive for occupational therapists. In the light of Estabrooks' (1997) experience, the terms *direct, indirect* and *persuasive* have been adopted for the definition of research utilisation being developed here.

It is recognised that, in order to understand research utilisation fully, it is necessary to take into account that this research use may be direct, indirect, or persuasive. In the case of occupational therapy, where there is limited robust research, most research use may be indirect. The language of McCurren's (1995) definition needs to be modified to ensure that this differentiation is explicit: 'a process in which the [valid] products of research are applied [directly, indirectly or persuasively] to verify current practice or to change current practice'. Therefore, a more complete definition of research utilisation can now be posited:

> **a process in which the valid products of research are applied directly, indirectly or persuasively to verify current practice or to change current practice.**
> (Bannigan, 2004, p. 282)

Now that we have arrived at a definition of research utilisation, the different facets of the definition can be unpacked to start to understand more clearly what research utilisation involves:

- It is a process;
- It involves making judgements about the rigour of research and practice;
- Sometimes change will be involved;
- It is a generic skill, and
- It is a macro skill.

What is involved in research utilisation?

Whether direct, indirect or persuasive, research utilisation involves a process; it is 'a course of action or proceeding' (*Concise Oxford Dictionary of Current English*, 1990, p. 951), never just a one-off action or task. This process:

- may not always be linear, for example, many of those involved perceive or experience barriers to this process;
- may be a composite of processes;
- in the case of indirect research utilisation, may involve cognitive processes rather than external physical actions.

Part of the process of research utilisation involves making a judgement about research findings. There are two aspects to this judgement: rigour and relevance. The rigour of research methodology has to be assessed because all research is subject to bias, which may have distorted the findings. If biased research findings are used in practice, it may be that the occupational therapist ends up doing more harm than good. The relevance of the findings also has to be considered. For example, a research study may be well conducted and have statistically signifi-cant findings but if the findings are not clinically significant they should not be applied to practice. The judgements made about research often govern whether the research is used at all or if it is used directly or indirectly.

If the judgement is that the research is rigorous and relevant, it is then necessary to consider the findings in relation to current practice. This may just involve verification or it may involve use, which could be direct or indirect. If direct use is the agreed course of action, this may require a process of planned change because research findings alone are not enough to change practice. Change involves a number of issues (Keep, 1998), such as resources (including time and people), readiness to change and, in order to bring these different aspects of the change process together, rigorous planning (Audit Commission, 2001). The issues involved in a process of change may also depend on the occupational therapist's role. For example, 'Administrators [i.e. managers] are responsible for creating an institutional climate that fosters and promotes research use whereas clinicians are responsible for the adaptation, implementation, and clinical evaluation of the research' (Funk *et al.*, 1995, p. 44).

An ability to use research findings is needed to improve or develop practice but the process of research utilisation does not rely on specialist clinical skills. Like communication, research utilisation is a generic skill that all professionals working in health and social care need to be able to use: it is not the province of any one professional group.

The skill of research utilisation is a composite of sub- or micro skills and relies on other skills, such as problem solving. Each aspect of the process requires different skills, for example, the initial stage of making a judgement about the quality of research is made up of a number of component skills, such as literature searching. Within each of these components there are also different micro skills, for example, finding information requires the ability to design and implement search strategies and to retrieve the literature identified. This in turn, involves knowing how to use a range of technologies:

- Electronic databases;
- The Internet;
- Citations; and
- Library facilities.

Models of research utilisation

Within health and social care settings, three approaches have evolved in response to the problem of the research–practice gap: diffusion, dissemination and implementation.

The diffusion model

Diffusion models perceive research use as a linear process and are predicated on the belief: publish and it will be used. In reality, serendipity, 'the faculty of making happy and unexpected discoveries by accident' (*Concise Oxford Dictionary of Current English*, 1990, p. 1105), describes what actually happens in the process of diffusion (see Figure 10.1). Even if an occupational therapist finds or hears a paper with relevant research findings there is no guarantee that she will then act on what she has read or heard to change or verify clinical practice.

The dissemination model

The dissemination model is a targeted approach (NHS Centre for Review and Dissemination, 2001) (see Figure 10.2) and a more active process than diffusion. It is predicated on the belief that if research findings are presented in accessible formats, such as guidelines to key stakeholders, they will be used. However, dissemination is limited by:

- the researcher's knowledge and understanding of the target audiences;
- resources – both financial and time – required to generate and market materials;
- a lack of incentive: researchers are rewarded for publishing in high-impact journals (Garfield, 1994) and so have little incentive to disseminate more widely; equally, those occupational therapists targeted in a dissemination strategy have little incentive to pass findings on to their colleagues; and
- a focus on raising awareness rather than using research findings.

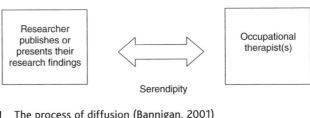

Figure 10.1 The process of diffusion (Bannigan, 2001)

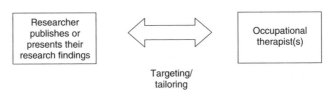

Figure 10.2 The process of dissemination (Bannigan, 2001)

Although a targeted approach increases the probability of research findings being shared, there is still an element of serendipity. And the question remains, does it change practice? Evidence suggests that dissemination alone does not impact on clinical practice (NHS Centre for Review and Dissemination, 1999).

The implementation model

As a result of the weakness of the dissemination model, a third approach to research use has emerged: implementation, which uses research findings to change practice (Mulhall and LeMay 1999) (see Figure 10.3). This 'is a more active process, which uses not only the message itself, but also organisational and behavioural tools that are sensitive to the constraints and opportunities identified by [occupational therapists] in identified settings' (Lomas 1993, p. 227).

A number of models, based on the dissemination model, proliferated in the nursing profession in the US in the 1970s, 1980s and 1990s. For example:

- The Nursing Child Assessment Satellite Training Project (NCAST) (Barnard and Hoehn, 1978);
- The Western Interstate Commission on Higher Education in Nursing Project (WICHE) (Krueger *et al.*, 1978);
- Conduct and Utilisation of Research in Nursing Project (CURN) (Horsley *et al.*, 1983);
- The linkage model (Crane, 1985a, b) and the Stetler-Marram model (Stetler, 1994).

All of these models of research utilisation appear to centre on some form of process. However, not all of them are about research utilisation per se. Some are about awareness raising (e.g. Barnard and Hoehn, 1978; Crane, 1985a, b), others are primarily about dissemination (e.g. Nolan *et al.*, 1994), while others aim to increase research utilisation but tend to follow the dissemination model and be focused on one set of research findings. Other difficulties with using these models are:

- they are nursing models, so they may not be applicable to occupational therapists;
- they were developed in America, so there may be cultural issues reducing their applicability in the UK or other countries; and
- they have not all been widely adopted and, since some of them have been in existence since the 1970s, it would appear that they have failed to capture the imagination.

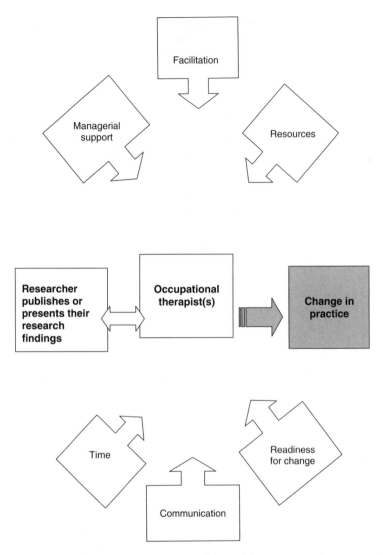

Figure 10.3 The process of implementation (adapted from Bryar and Bannigan, 2003, p. 69)

Research utilisation is still a general concern in the nursing literature, which implies that the use of these models has not yet had a lasting impact on research utilisation. It also suggests that, since the dissemination models used in nursing appear to have been ineffective in increasing the use of research findings in practice, the dissemination model itself may have limitations in relation to increasing the use of research findings.

Fostering the use of research findings

A total of 48 studies of interventions to increase the use of research findings have been identified (Bannigan, 2004). Identifying studies was extremely difficult because, as has already been highlighted, there is no standard nomenclature for research utilisation. Most of the research identified had been conducted by the nursing profession, although there were some studies by therapists, including occupational therapists (e.g. Jaramazovic and Curtin, 2000) and physiotherapists (e.g. Turner and Whitfield, 1997), and there was limited research in the field of medicine. However, doctors have tended to be involved in larger evaluation studies of discrete projects, such as FACTS (Munro *et al.*, 1995) or PACE (Dunning *et al.*, 1998). Many of the 48 studies were evaluations rather than formal research projects and the evaluation either tended not to be the priority or appeared to be a secondary aim, for example ASPIRE (Hollis and Foy, 2001). The projects were focused on the intervention and/or achieving changes in practice. Evaluating what changes occurred seems to have been in the background, if considered at all.

The evaluation studies tended to use a before-and-after methodology, along the lines of the dissemination model (see Figure 10.2 above). That is, specific research findings are targeted at the professionals and a before-and-after study is used to assess change in clinical practice. The measures used were clinical measures, such as lung function (Shah *et al.*, 2001) or treatment threshold for systolic hypertension (Cranney *et al.*, 1999). In these studies, the focus is on strong research evidence and not on transferable research utilisation skills. It is likely that the interventions studied neither inculcated nor assessed the ability of the professionals involved to generalise research utilisation skills to other research findings. Obviously, it is only possible to speculate about this because data were not collected on research use in these studies.

Many of the evaluations made use of questionnaires designed for the particular study. Generally, the development of these questionnaires involved little or no reliability and validity testing and did not take into account other studies or previous research. For example, in the development of the ACE pre-workshop/post-workshop questionnaires, Richardson and Jerosch-Herold (1998) used the Critical Appraisal Skills Programme workshop evaluation pre-workshop questionnaire but no other studies or tools.

Some studies were about doing research rather than using research, for example, Bostrom *et al.* (1989), while others focused on a subskill such as searching, for example, Michaud *et al.* (1996). Overall, in terms of quality, many of the studies lacked rigour. There was poor reporting so that where reliability and validity were referred to there was often not enough information to judge this. Despite these weaknesses, 18 measures were identified where reliability and validity had been considered in the development of a questionnaire, but none was sufficiently reliable and valid to be used in a study to evaluate an intervention without further development (Bannigan, 2004). As with the models developed by the nursing profession in the US (above), this indicates that a large number of studies have been conducted using the dissemination model but there does not appear to have been a corresponding impact on long-term research utilisation by the professionals involved.

Measures of research utilisation

There has not been a lack of attention to measurement on the part of researchers studying research utilisation. The number of measures identified clearly shows that some attention has been paid to measurement in this field. The problem is a lack of reference to previous research, resulting in a lack of coherence in relation to measurement in research utilisation. For example, authors refer to 'the' literature when developing scales (e.g. Upton and Lewis, 1998) but it is not clear what this literature was or how it was used. The reference lists often indicate that very little of the available literature has actually been considered.

Without robust measurement, it is not possible to design or conduct the rigorous studies that are needed to evaluate interventions, such as the Turnkey manual, which was developed to increase the use of research by allied health professionals, including occupational therapists (Bannigan, 2004). For example, a body of research is needed to provide the data for calculating sample sizes, particularly for studies that need to make use of intra-cluster correlation coefficients. Evans and Haines (2000) have commented there is a need to 'address the imbalance between the growing volume of literature on the theory of evidence-practice and the lack of material on implementation based on real world experience' (p. xvii). Without the concomitant development of the measures needed to evaluate interventions, much of this work may be of limited value because it will not be possible to generalise findings.

Reliable and valid measures are needed to evaluate research utilisation interventions as they are developed. Although some reliable and valid measures can be identified, few have been tested very widely. McDowell and Newell (1996) suggested that construct validity is needed to develop a robust measure. The features of good studies of construct validity are:

- a clear statement of hypotheses with justification of why they are the most relevant;
- testing the stated hypotheses;
- trying to disprove the hypothesis that the method measures something other than its stated purpose;

- assessing construct validity through convergent validity (that uses correlational evidence), factorial validity or discriminant validity (that uses group differences or discriminant evidence).

Construct validity is dependent on a coherent understanding of a construct. Estabrooks (1997) concluded that the lack of definition and coherence is:

> an indication that we do not yet have a critical mass of researchers working cohesively on the problem in the area. Until such time as we do have such debates we cannot be confident that we are progressing satisfactorily toward better science in the field.
>
> (Estabrooks, 1997, p. 137)

The experience of researching this field from an allied health perspective resonates strongly with this observation (Bannigan, 2004). The field is so disparate and ghettoised in the professions that links between researchers do not form in order for networks to develop to facilitate the debates that Estabrooks (1997) has indicated are missing. This situation is likely to persist until researchers move out of the segregated groups of their own profession and start tackling the problem together.

A way forward

Research utilisation is a complex problem and 'successful research implementation is a highly complex and interdisciplinary undertaking' (Closs and Cheater, 1994, pp. 770–1).

There is a reasonable human desire to reduce the problem into a simpler form, hence the models of diffusion and dissemination. However, there are 'complex problems involved in moving research findings into practice' (Tornquist et al., 1995, p. 106) and an assessment of skills cannot be decontextualised (Rodgers, 1994). This means that a range of aspects needs to be considered, such as the:

- micro skills involved;
- barriers;
- infrastructure (as an indication of the organisational culture) within which the individual is operating; and
- individual's attitude.

Taken together with the five components of evidence-based practice described on page 191, these aspects provide an overview of an individual's ability to use research. Without capturing data about all these issues, it may be that indirect research use will not be identified in the same way as direct research use. Equally, without a measure of attitude an individual may seem antithetic to the use of research-based knowledge when, in fact, they are not hostile but are experiencing other problems such as a lack of skills or the constraints of resources, culture or the nature of research. No one aspect will provide a complete overview of research utilisation, which suggests that any measure of research utilisation may need to be a profile of measures.

This exploration of the concept of research utilisation illustrates the complexity of the problem.

It feels as if the time has come to face this reality, to stop running away from these complexities and to recognise that research utilisation is a complex problem without a simple solution. Instead of trying to find simple answers, all involved need to embrace the complexity. A guiding principle to bear in mind when thinking about this paraphrases the words of the journalist, *H.L. Mencken*: 'For every complex problem, there is a simple solution, and . . . it's wrong.' However, human beings like simple solutions because they are easy. It is often only when you get inside a complex issue that you realise just how complex it is, and this can be disabling. With so many different facets to the problem, and working in an ever-changing environment such as the NHS, with the potential for many problems (e.g. barriers), the task could be overwhelming. The tension is that, if there is a sincere belief that the use of research findings improves the quality of patient care, something has to be done to increase research use although we have exhausted the simple solutions. The challenge for those working in this field is to reconcile the complexity issue so that movement rather than inertia is created.

It seems that much of the thinking and work surrounding research utilisation is mechanistic. Research use as a process tends to be atomised; that is, researchers focus on one aspect in isolation from or with limited reference to the bigger picture. The issue of complexity is avoided because complexity presents a problem to the method of science (Checkland, 1999). This seems to be at the root of why this knowledge base is still in an embryonic state. For example, research into barriers to research utilisation has, until recently, only been replicated in various settings with different professional groups, with little reference to the wider field. There has also been little reported in the way of the activity to overcome the barriers. This focus on individual professional groups, despite research utilisation being a generic skill, is another way in which the field is atomised.

The mechanistic worldview

The atomising of a question is indicative of a mechanistic worldview. Mechanism is typical of conventional scientific method:

> One aspect of the mechanistic worldview that they have paid particular atten-
> tion to is reductionism (narrowing attention to linear, causal relationships
> between variables, thereby failing to see that these relationships can only be
> adequately understood as aspects of the operation of wider systems). Reduc-
> tionism follows on logically from mechanism in that, if someone believes that
> systems are no more than the sum of their parts, it makes sense to decompose
> them into those parts to increase understanding.
>
> (Midgley, 2000, p. 39)

This mode of thinking, when it is incorporated into research methodology, involves three stages:

1. Dissect conceptually/physically.
2. Learn the properties/behaviour of the separate parts.
3. From the properties of the parts, deduce the properties/behaviour of the whole. (Skyttner, 1996, p. 10)

This approach to research runs into difficulties when researchers are faced with highly complex, real-world problems set in a social context, such as research utilisation.

Complexity science

If complexity is at the heart of the problem, complexity science may offer solutions. Complexity science, or chaos theory, is gaining credence in health and social care. In 2001 the *British Medical Journal* ran a series of articles on complexity science (Fraser and Greenhalgh, 2001; Plsek and Greenhalgh, 2001; Plsek and Wilson, 2001; Wilson *et al.*, 2001). Chaos and complexity theorists 'argue that it is simply not possible to plan with such certainty' (Midgely, 2000, p. 122) and 'use new ideas in mathematics to show that much of what happens, far from being inher-ently predictable, is actually *un*predictable' (Midgely, 2000, p. 2). The difficulty with the science of complexity is that it is 'a subject that's still so new and so wide-ranging that nobody knows quite how to define it, or even where its boundaries lie . . . complexity research is trying to grapple with questions that defy all the conventional categories' (Waldrop, 1992: 9). So, while complexity science may have potential, what is most useful in these theories is the focus on systems. This leads into an exploration of systems thinking.

Systems thinking

Systems thinking is a philosophical position that has answered some of the con-cerns posed by the mechanistic worldview, where:

systems thinking focuses on the feedback relationships between the thing being studied and the other parts of the system. Therefore instead of isolating smaller and smaller parts of a system, systems thinking involves a broader view, looking at larger and larger numbers of interactions. In this way, systems thinking creates a better understanding of the big picture.

(Aronson, 2003, p. 1)

In systems thinking, the concept of *system* embodies the notion of a collection of elements connected together to form a whole. 'Systems thinking complements scientific method by dealing with such complexities' (UK Systems Society, 2003). Many theories have developed based on systems thinking, for example, the hierarchy of systems complexity and the Gaia hypothesis. It is beyond the scope of this discussion to explore these in detail but there is a basic idea and some key features to systems thinking that characterise all of these theoretical interpretations and which are explained below.

The basic idea of systems thinking, in contrast to mechanistic thinking, is that:

Systems thinking expands the focus of the observer, whereas analytical thinking reduces it. In other words, analysis looks into things, synthesis looks out of them. This attitude of systems is often called expansionism, an alternative to classic reductionism. Whereas analytical thinking concentrates on static and structural properties, systems thinking concentrates on the function and behaviour of whole systems. Analysis gives description and knowledge; systems thinking gives explanation and understanding. With its emphasis on variation and multiplicity, rather than statistically ensured regularities, systems thinking belongs to the holistic tradition of ideas.

(Skyttner, 1996, p. 21)

Systems thinking has two key features: emergence and hierarchy, and communication and control (Checkland, 1999). Other features include interdisciplinarity and pluralism. Emergence and hierarchy refer to holism, which involves taking 'seriously the idea of a whole entity which may exhibit properties as a single whole ("emergent properties"), properties which have no meaning in terms of the parts of the whole' (Checkland and Scholes, 1990, p. 25).

To do systems thinking is to set some constructed abstract wholes (often called 'systems models') against the perceived real world in order to learn about it. The purpose of doing this may range from engineering (in the broad sense of the word) some part of the world perceived as a system to seeking insight or illumination.

(Checkland and Scholes, 1990, p. 25)

Communication and control refer to the idea that 'in any hierarchy of open systems, maintenance of the hierarchy will entail a set of processes in which there is communication of information for the purposes of regulation or control' (Checkland, 1999, p. 83). Together, emergence and hierarchy and communication and control 'generate the image or metaphor of the adaptive whole which may be able to survive in a changing environment' (Checkland and Scholes, 1990, p. 19).

Systems thinking is interdisciplinary, having moved away from the conventional scientific view of specialisation and compartmentalisation (Skyttner, 1996). It also tends to be 'more ethical, less philosophical' (Skyttner, 1996, p. 23) in focus and pluralist in nature, that is, it draws on a wide range of theories and methods so that they are not seen as competing. This means that systems theorists 'can accept a plurality of theories flowing into methodology, and hence a wide variety of methods may be seen as legitimate' (Midgely, 2000, p. 171).

An obvious danger inherent in this approach to thinking about the world is arrogance. How can any researcher or research team be truly holistic? Even if they believe that they have been, it is likely that they will have missed aspects of the whole system. Another danger is that studies become unwieldy in their attempt to deal with the whole. This means that, while the application of systems thinking is useful in researching complex problems, it needs to be used with a degree of humility. Researchers using systems thinking need to recognise that they cannot understand or explain everything. In some ways this takes us back to the start of this philosophical musing: if systems thinking is only capable of looking at part of the whole, surely it is of little more use than the mechanistic approach of conventional science? This is not necessarily the case if the boundary concept is taken on board.

The boundary concept

Boundary judgements are a practical way of thinking about complexity. A boundary 'is a distinction made by an observer which marks the difference between an entity he takes to be a system and its environment' (Checkland, 1999, p. 312). The boundary concept is central to systems thinking because:

> once we acknowledge that no view of the world can ever be comprehensive, the boundary concept becomes crucial. Where exactly boundaries are constructed, and what the values are that guide the construction, will determine how issues are seen and what actions will be taken.
>
> (Midgely, 2000, p. 36)

It is:

> the motivation of systems thinkers to be as comprehensive as possible in their analyses. As it is impossible for any analysis to be totally comprehensive, this leads on to a consideration of boundary judgement: Judgements about what is to be included or excluded from analyses.
>
> (Midgely, 2000, p. 33)

It is important to note that:

> a boundary does not simply mark what is included within it. It also marks what is excluded. However, for there to be any awareness of what is excluded, a second boundary must be apparent . . . Everything is distinguished from that which it is not, and that which it is not comes to be distinguished in turn with references to another boundary.
>
> (Midgely, 2000, pp. 36–7)

When making boundary judgements 'It is necessary to explore different possible boundary judgements in order to optimise the inclusion of information in analyses' (Midgely, 2000, p. 38) and recognise that 'boundary judgements and values are intimately connected' (Midgely, 2000, p. 136). This means that researchers have to find a way to make choices but they have to be careful not to disempower other key stakeholders. This entails considering who is involved, what values you are using and whether other groups will be marginalised. It is also possible to assess which choice to make and how the choice was made through boundary critique. This critical scrutiny is vital because of the value judgements involved in boundary judgement (Midgely, 2000).

Using systems thinking to make sense of research utilisation

The focus of this chapter is research utilisation. It has been shown that the way in which the field has been researched to date has not allowed the concept to develop sufficiently. This appears to be due to the need to simplify the problem and so reduce it into smaller parts, which is a characteristic of mechanistic thinking. However, there are other ways of thinking about the world, such as systems thinking. The application of systems thinking, and branches within it such as complexity science, allows a more holistic approach to the evaluation of research utilisation. If researchers in the field take on board these ideas, they may provide a way of coping with the complexity that has beset studies to date. It would also signal a move away from reliance on the dissemination model. These ideas need to be developed further but what they offer is an opportunity to think differently about the problem.

This idea is not without precedent. Goode *et al.* (1987) used systems theory to depict the process of using research-based knowledge in clinical practice. Systems thinking may or may not prove to be helpful in thinking about methodology, but at least it provides an alternative to a methodology that has driven this field of research into a rut.

In a practice setting, a clinical specialist given the responsibility of ensuring that some recently published research findings are implemented in practice would behave very differently if she allowed systems thinking to influence her work rather than the dissemination model (Box 10.1).

Box 10.1: Case example

A consultant occupational therapist leading a stroke rehabilitation service has to respond to a recent Cochrane review, published by Legg *et al.*, 2006, which found that 'Patients who receive occupational therapy interventions are less likely to deteriorate and are more likely to be independent in their ability to perform personal activities of daily living' (p. 1).

Following the dissemination model, the therapist would make sure that a summary of the review's findings reached all the relevant people in the organisation. This summary may involve a dissemination conference and/or a user-friendly précis. Once this had been done, she could assume that those who received this summary would then act on it to change their practice.

Using systems thinking, the therapist would adopt a very different approach. The starting point would still be the research findings but she would think carefully about how they related to the different people in the organisation. This could involve facilitating discussions about the research findings and their implications for practice, which would then shape what she does next. This is because she would recognise that the response of the key stakeholders to the findings will shape how the organisation responds. While she may draw on change management theory to inform this work, what she does will depend on the individuals involved and the needs of the organisation, recognising that the different parts are all interrelated.

Another approach that the occupational therapist could use is action research, which enables 'practitioners, managers and researchers to make sense of problems in service delivery and in promoting initiatives for change and improvement' (Hart and Bond, 1995, p. 3). Whatever processes the consultant therapist uses with her team, these processes will be different the next time she has to implement research findings. This is because, using systems thinking, she would complete a feedback loop based on this experience. While she may learn useful rules of thumb, it would not be possible to develop a rubric that she could follow for future scenarios. For example, she may learn about the importance of facilitating communication with and between key stakeholders but not a mechanism that can be used to communicate with all stakeholders whenever she has to implement research findings. This is because people will respond differently to change at different times; organisations change and having to approach a task for the second time means the stakeholders will have skills and expectations that they may not have had when they first engaged with research utilisation.

The need for surrogate end points

Rogers (1995) described how, when diffusion researchers became an 'invisible college', they began to limit unnecessarily the ways in which they went about studying the diffusion of innovations, and claimed that such standardisation of approaches constrains the intellectual progress of diffusion research. This appears to be what has happened in relation to research on research utilisation. There is no clear justification for using the dissemination model but it seems to have become standard practice.

The reason for the widespread adoption of the dissemination model may be related to the belief that surrogate end points (or interim measures) should not be used in health services research. The assumption is made that the only important outcome for a health service is a clinical outcome, that is, something that has a direct and meaningful impact on patient care. Usually, this assumption would make inherent sense: while there is a place for 'blue skies' research, it is accepted that funds for health services research should be used for studies that are directly relevant to patient care. Using these criteria, research utilisation skills are a surrogate end point and so their use is invalidated.

While it is not the norm to use surrogate end points in health services research, it can be argued that they are needed in this field because change is so difficult to achieve and to measure. If clinical change continues to be regarded as the only acceptable measure, it could be that an intervention which moves clinicians part way along the continuum of research use would be discounted. This is because the effect would not be detected since relevant data were not collected. However, the use of surrogate end points actually represents a realistic view of the complexity of change and is a more theoretically appropriate way of researching research utilisation, based on the nature of change.

The use of surrogate end points could serve two purposes: detecting effects not identified by solely focusing on clinical change, and providing a source of motivation for staff. If change is difficult to achieve, those engaged in the process are more likely to continue if they can see that they are progressing along a continuum towards the long-term aim of improving patient care; therefore, monitoring incremental steps is an important tool for motivating further change.

This type of measure may also be the only way to measure the indirect use of research, which is a causal factor in overall research utilisation, as described above. Therefore, measures of research utilisation are not meaningless interim measures but recognise that there is a need to be realistic about the nature of change, that it is helpful to provide an indication of performance along the continuum and that context must be taken into account. There needs to be wider recognition that surrogate end points are appropriate so that research using surrogate end points is funded and more coherence in the field is promoted.

Rogers (1995) suggested that we do not need more of the same research on research utilisation. This means that there is a need to rethink the design of future studies so that they are not necessarily based on the dissemination model. The challenge for research utilisation scholars of the future is to move beyond methods based on the dissemination model, to recognise the shortcomings and limitations of these methods and to broaden their conceptions of research utilisation. Systems thinking, with its emphasis on plurality, may be one means by which researchers studying research utilisation can start to think outside the box. This may offer solutions or ways forward needed to advance knowledge in the field.

There also needs to be a shift in focus so that interventions rather than barriers are the focus of research. Therapists clearly perceive and/or experience barriers to research utilisation but research in this area needs to be put on hold so that interventions can be developed to overcome them. More barriers research may refine what we know of the barriers experienced by occupational therapists but it does not enable therapists to translate their enthusiasm into action. There is more urgency for interventions to be developed and evaluated that enable practitioners to use research findings in everyday practice.

Summary

This chapter has demonstrated that research utilisation is still a nascent subject; a critical review of the state of the art has indicated that there is a lack of definition, interdisciplinary research and coherence in the field. Systems thinking, including the concept of boundaries, has been explored as a means of researching this complex concept. It may also provide a way forward for interdisciplinary working, and so establish this emerging subject. There is a need to face up to the complexity of research utilisation but it should be remembered that, if research utilisation does not happen, the time and money invested in health services research is being wasted. Perhaps this expenditure should stop? Or perhaps spending on the development aspect of research and development should be increased? If there are no further funds available, the amount spent on research and development should be split 50-50 between the conduct and implementation of research projects.

Occupational therapists clearly perceive and/or experience barriers to research utilisation. There has been a focus on barriers research but this should be put on hold so that interventions to overcome the barriers can be developed. The focus should shift to interventions, and these interventions should be rigorously evaluated. This means that a reliable and valid measure, or profile of measures, of research utilisation needs to be developed so that there are robust tools available to evaluate interventions. Researchers need to explore more creative ways of looking at the problem of research utilisation and may find that systems thinking offers a valid alternative to the dissemination model. When there is more coherence in knowledge gathering about research use, it may increase the likelihood of knowledge application in relation to research use and so reduce the research–practice gap experienced by occupational therapists.

References

Aronson, D. (2003) Targeted innovation using systems thinking to increase the benefits of innovation efforts, http://www.thinking.net/systems_thinking/systems_thinking.html (25 February 2003).

Audit Commission (2001) *Change Here! Managing Change to Improve Local Services*, Audit Commission, London.

Bannigan, K. (2001) Annual AOTMH Lecture 2001: Sharing the evidence for mental health occupational therapy practice. *Mental Health OT*, **6**(2), 4–9.

Bannigan, K. (2004) Increasing the use of research findings in four allied health professions (unpublished PhD thesis), School of Nursing, University of Hull, Hull.

Barnard, K.E. and Hoehn, R.E. (1978) *Nursing Child Assessment Satellite Training* (final report), **DHEW**, Division of Nursing, Hyattsville, MD.

Bostrom, A.C., Malnight, M., MacDougall, J. and Hargis, D (1989) Staff nurses' attitudes toward nursing research: a descriptive survey. *Journal of Advanced Nursing*, **14**, 915–22.

Carter, D. (1996) Barriers to the implementation of research findings in practice *Nurse Researcher*, **4**(2), 30–40.

Checkland, P. (1999) *Systems Thinking, Systems Practice*, John Wiley & Sons, Chichester, UK.

Checkland, P. and Scholes, J. (1990) *Soft Systems Methodology in Action*, John Wiley & Sons, Chichester, UK.

Closs, S.J. and Cheater, F.M. (1994) Utilisation of nursing research: culture, interest and support. *Journal of Advanced Nursing*, **19**, 762–73.

Closs, S.J. and Lewin, B.J.P. (1998) Perceived barriers to research utilisation: a survey of four therapies *British Journal of Therapy and Rehabilitation*, **5**(3), 151–5.

College of Occupational Therapists (2005) *College of Occupational Therapists Code of Ethics and Professional Conduct*, College of Occupational Therapists, London.

Concise Oxford Dictionary of Current English 8th edition (1990) Oxford University Press, Oxford.

Crane, J. (1985a) Research utilisation: theoretical perspectives. *Western Journal of Nursing Research*, **7**, 261–8.

Crane, J. (1985b) Research utilisation: nursing models. *Western Journal of Nursing Research*, **7**, 494–7.

Cranney, M., Barton, S. and Walley, T. (1999) Addressing barriers to change: an RCT practice-based education to improve the management of hypertension in the elderly. *British Journal of General Practice*, **49**, 522–6.

Crosswaite, C. and Curtice, L. (1994) Disseminating research results: the challenge of bridging the gap between health research and health action. *Health Promotion International*, **9**(4), 289–96.

Dawes, M., Summerskill, W., Glasziou, P., Cartabellotta, A., Martin, J., Hopayian, K., Porzolt, F., Burls, A. and Osborne, J. (2005) Sicily statement on evidence-based practice. *BMC Medical Education* **5**, 1, doi: 10.1186/1472-6920-5-1, http://www.biomedcentral.com/1472–6920/5/1 (18 February 2005).

Department of Health (n.d.) www.dh.gov.uk (Ten key skills for allied health professionals).

Department of Health (2000) *The NHS Plan*, HMSO, Norwich.

Dunning, M., Abi-Aad, G., Gilbert, D., Hutton, H. and Brown, C. (1998) *Experience, Evidence and Everyday Practice: Creating Systems for Delivering Effective Health Care*, King's Fund, London.

Enderby, P., Ilott, I. and Newham, D. (1998) Foreword, in *Evidence-Based Healthcare: A Practical Guide for Therapists* (eds T. Bury and J. Mead), Butterworth-Heinemann, Oxford, pp. vii–viii.

Estabrooks, C.A. (1997) Research utilisation in nursing: an examination of formal structure and influencing factors (unpublished PhD thesis), University of Alberta, Edmonton, Alberta, Canada.

Evans, D. and Haines, A. (eds) (2000) *Implementing Evidence-Based Changes in Healthcare*, Radcliffe Medical Press, Abingdon, UK.

Fraser, S.W. and Greenhalgh, T. (2001) Complexity science: coping with complexity, educating for capability. *British Medical Journal*, **323**, 799–803.

Funk, S.G., Champagne, M.T., Tornquist, E.M. and Wiese, R.A. (1995) Administrators' views on barriers to research utilisation. *Applied Nursing Research*, **8**(1), 44–9.

Garfield, E. (1994) The impact factor. *Current Contents* 20 June 1994, http://www.isinet.com/isi/hot/essays/journalcitationreports/7.html (26 March 2003).

Goode, C.J., Lovett, M.K., Hayes, J.E. and Butcher, L.A. (1987) Use of research-based knowledge in clinical practice *Journal of Nursing Administration*, **17**(12), 11–18.

Grimshaw, J.M. and Thomson, M.A. (1998) What have new efforts to change professional practice achieved? *Journal of the Royal Society of Medicine* Supplement, **35**(91), 20–5.

Hart, E. and Bond, M. (1995) *Action Research for Health and Social Care: A Guide to Practice*, Open Univeristy Press, Buckingham, UK.

Hollis, S. and Foy, R. (2001) *ASPIRE Action to Support Practice Implementing Research Evidence* (draft report), Lancaster University, Lancaster, UK.

Horsley, J., Crane, J., Crabtree, M. and Wood, D. (1983) *Using Research to Improve Nursing Practice: A Guide*, Grune & Stratton, New York.

Ilott, I. and White, E. (2001) College of Occupational Therapists' research and development strategic vision and action plan. *British Journal of Occupational Therapy*, **64**(6), 270–7.

Jaramazovic, E. and Curtin, M. (2000) Occupational therapy and the use of evidence-based practice. *British Journal of Occupational Therapy*, **64**(5), 214–22.

Keep, J. (1998) Change management, in *Evidence-Based Healthcare: A Practical Guide for Therapists* (eds T. Bury and J. Mead), Butterworth-Heinemann, Oxford, pp. 44–65.

Kirk, S. (1998) The NHS research and development strategy, in *Research and Development for the NHS: Evidence, Evaluation and Effectiveness*, 2nd edn (eds M. Baker and S. Kirk), Radcliffe Medical Press, Oxford, UK, pp. 1–8.

Krueger, J., Nelson, A. and Wolanin, M. (1978) *Nursing Research: Development, Collaboration and Utilisation*, Aspen, Germantown, MD.

Larsen, J. (1980) Knowledge utilization. What is it? *Knowledge: Creation, Diffusion, Utilization*, **1**, 421–44.

Legg, L.A., Drummond, A.E. and Langhorne, P. (2006) Occupational therapy for patients with problems in activities of daily living after stroke. *Cochrane Database of Systematic Reviews* 2006, Issue 4. Art. No.: CD003585. DOI: 10.1002/14651858. CD003585.pub2.

Lomas, J. (1993) Diffusion, dissemination, and implementation: who should do what? *Annals New York Academy of Sciences*, **703**, 226–37.

McCurren, C.D. (1995) Research utilisation: meeting the challenge. *Geriatric Nursing*, **16**, 132–5.

McDowell, I. and Newell, C. (1996) *Measuring Health: A Guide to Rating Scales and Questionnaires*, 2nd edn, Oxford University Press, New York.

Metcalfe, C.M., Lewin, R., Wisher, S., Perry, S., Bannigan, K. and Klaber Moffet, J. (2001) Barriers to implementing the evidence base in four NHS therapies: dietitians, occupational therapists, physiotherapists, speech and language therapists. *Physiotherapy*, **87**(8), 433–41.

Michaud, G.C., McGowan, J.L., van der Jagt, R.H., Dugan, A.K. and Tugwell, P. (1996) The introduction of evidence-based medicine as a component of daily practice. *Bulletin of the Medical Library Association*, **84**(4), 478–81.

Midgley, G. (2000) *Systemic Intervention: Philosophy, Methodology and Practice*, Kluwer Academic/Plenum Publishers, New York.

Mulhall, A. and Le May, A. (eds) (1999) *Nursing Research Dissemination and Implementation*, Churchill Livingstone, Edinburgh.

Munro, J., Eve, R., Golton, I., Hodgkin, P. and Musson, G. (1995) Facing the FACTS. *Health Service Journal*, 5 October, 26–7.

NHS Centre for Reviews and Dissemination (1999) Getting evidence into practice. *Effective Health Care*, **5**(1), Royal Society of Medicine Press, London.

NHS Centre for Reviews and Dissemination (2001) Dissemination, http://www.york. ac.uk/inst/crd/dissinfo.htm (26 March 2001).

Nolan, M.T., Larson, E., McGuire, D., Hill, M.N. and Haller, K. (1994) A review of approaches to integrating research and practice. *Applied Nursing Research*, **7**, 199–207.

Plsek, P.E. and Greenhalgh, T. (2001) Complexity science: the challenge of complexity in health care. *British Medical Journal*, **323**, 625–8.

Plsek, P.E. and Wilson, T. (2001) Complexity science: complexity, leadership, and management in healthcare organisations. *British Medical Journal*, **323**, 746–9.

Pollock, A.S., Legg, L., Langhorne, P. and Sellars, C. (2000) Barriers to achieving evidence-based stroke rehabilitation. *Clinical Rehabilitation*, **14**, 611–17.

Richardson, B. and Jerosch-Herold, C. (1998) Appraisal of clinical effectiveness: an ACE approach to promoting evidence-based therapy. *Journal of Clinical Effectiveness*, **3**(4), 146–50.

Rodgers, S. (1994) An exploratory study of research utilisation by nurses in general medical and surgical wards. *Journal of Advanced Nursing*, **20**, 904–11.

Rogers, E.M. (1995) *Diffusion of Innovations*, 4th edn, Free Press, New York.

Rosenberg, W. and Donald, A. (1995) Evidence based medicine: an approach to clinical problem solving. *British Medical Journal*, **310**, 1122–6.

Sackett, D.L., Richardson, W.S., Rosenberg, W. and Haynes, B.R. (1997) *Evidence-Based Medicine: How to Practice and Teach EBM*, Churchill Livingstone, New York.

Sackett, D.L., Richardson, W.S., Rosenberg, W. and Haynes, B.R. (2000) *Evidence-Based Medicine: How to Practice and Teach EBM*, 2nd edn, Churchill Livingstone, New York.

Shah, S., Peat, J.K., Mazurski, E.J., Sindhusake, D., Bruce, C., Henry, R.L. and Gibson, P.G. (2001) Effect of peer-led programme for asthma education in adolescents: cluster randomised controlled trial. *British Medical Journal*, **322**, 583–5.

Skyttner, L. (1996) *General Systems Theory: An Introduction*, Macmillan, London.

Stetler, C.B. (1994) Refinement of the Stetler/Marram model for application of research findings to practice. *Nursing Outlook*, **42**, 15–25.

Steultjens, E.M.J., Dekker, J., Bouter, L.M., van Schaardenberg, D., van Kuyk. M.A.H. and van den Ende, C.H.M. (2004) Occupational therapy for rheumatoid arthritis. *Cochrane Database of Systematic Reviews* 2004, Issue 1. Art No: CD003114 DOI: 10.1002/14651858.CD003114.pub2.

Straus, S.E., Richardson, W.S., Glasziou, P. and Haynes, R.B. (2005) *Evidence-Based Medicine: How to Practice and Teach EBM*, 3rd edn, Elsevier Churchill Livingstone, Edinburgh.

Sutherland, L. (2001) Welcome and opening remarks, in *Proceedings of the Conference on Evidence Based Decision Making: How to Keep Score?* (HTA Initiative #3), Alberta Heritage Foundation for Medical Research, Alberta, Canada, p. 3.

Tornquist, E.M., Funk, S.G. and Champagne, M.T. (1995) Research utilisation: reconnecting research and practice. *AACN Clinical Issues*, **6**(1), 105–9.

Turner, P. and Whitfield, T.W.A. (1997) Physiotherapists' use of evidence-based practice: a cross national study. *Physiotherapy Research International*, **2**(1), 17–29.

UK Systems Society (2003) UKSS information page, http://www.hebel.co.uk/UKSS/information.htm (12 April 2003).

Upton, D. (1999) Clinical effectiveness and EBP 2: attitudes of health care professionals. *British Journal of Therapy and Rehabilitation*, **6**(1), 26–30.

Upton, D. and Lewis, B. (1998) Clinical effectiveness and EBP: design of a questionnaire. *British Journal of Therapy and Rehabilitation*, **5**(12), 647–50.

Waldrop, M.W. (1992) *Complexity: The Emerging Science at the Edge of Order and Chaos*, Simon & Schuster, New York.

Wilson, T., Holt, T. and Greenhalgh, T. (2001) Complexity science: complexity and clinical care. *British Medical Journal*, **323**, 685–8.

Index